S0-ART-865

Perinatal
Patient
Education

David Graham

Perinatal Patient Education

A PRACTICAL GUIDE WITH EDUCATION HANDOUTS FOR PATIENTS

Margaret Comerford Freda, EdD, RN, CHES, FAAN

Associate Professor
Department of Obstetrics & Gynecology
and Women's Health

Albert Einstein College of Medicine,
Montefiore Medical Center
Bronx, New York

Editor
MCN: The American Journal
of Maternal-Child Nursing

LIPPINCOTT WILLIAMS & WILKINS
A **Wolters Kluwer** Company

Philadelphia • Baltimore • New York • London
Buenos Aires • Hong Kong • Sydney • Tokyo

Acquisitions Editor: Jennifer Brogan
Assistant Editor: Susan Barta Rainey
Senior Production Editor: Sandra Cherrey Scheinin
Senior Production Manager: Helen Ewan
Design Coordinator: Doug Smock
Manufacturing Manager: William Alberti
Indexer: Gaye Tarallo
Printer: Victor Graphics

Copyright © 2002 by Lippincott Williams & Wilkins. All rights reserved. This book is protected by copyright. No part of it may be reproduced, stored in a retrieval system or transmitted, in any form or by any means—electronic, mechanical, photocopy, recording, or otherwise—without prior written permission of the publisher, except for patient education handouts, which may be copied for clinical use but may not be copied for resale purposes, and for brief quotations embodied in critical articles and reviews and testing and evaluation materials provided by publisher to instructors whose schools have adopted its accompanying textbook. Printed in the United States of America. For information write Lippincott Williams & Wilkins, 530 Walnut Street, Philadelphia, PA 19106.

Materials appearing in this book prepared by individuals as part of their official duties as U.S. Government employees are not covered by the above-mentioned copyright.

9 8 7 6 5 4 3 2 1

Library of Congress Cataloging-in Publication Data

Freda, Margaret Comerford.
    Perinatal patient education : a practical guide with education handouts for patients /
  Margaret Comerford Freda.
      p. cm.
    Includes bibliographical references and index.
    ISBN 0-7817-3233-6 (alk. paper)
      1. Prenatal care--Study and teaching. 2. patient eduction. 3. Maternity nursing I. Title.

RG973.F74 2002
618.2'4--DC21

                                                          2002019782

Care has been taken to confirm the accuracy of the information presented and to describe generally accepted practices. However, the authors, editors, and publisher are not responsible for errors or omissions or for any consequences from application of the information in this book and make no warranty, express or implied, with respect to the content of the publication.

The authors, editors, and publisher have exerted every effort to ensure that drug selection and dosage set forth in this text are in accordance with the current recommendations and practice at the time of publication. However, in view of ongoing research, changes in government regulations, and the constant flow of information relating to drug therapy and drug reactions, the reader is urged to check the package insert for each drug for any change in indications and dosage and for added warnings and precautions. This is particularly important when the recommended agent is a new or infrequently employed drug.

Some drugs and medical devices presented in this publication have Food and Drug Administration (FDA) clearance for limited use in restricted research settings. It is the responsibility of the health care provider to ascertain the FDA status of each drug or device planned for use in his or her clinical practice.

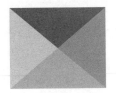

Preface

Welcome to my book! I've wanted to write this book for a very long time, and it's a real privilege for me to finally see this come to fruition. I think I realized that patient education was my favorite part of nursing back when I was in my diploma nursing school in the 1960s. Even then, when I was trying desperately to figure out how to please my instructor, keep the IV running properly, and use the correct number of towels for the bed bath (and usually doing at least two of those things wrong), it was always fun for me to answer my patients' questions and help them understand a little more about their treatment or diagnosis.

As the years went by, and I graduated and then became a labor and delivery nurse, my fascination grew with how little the average woman knew about how her body works and what would happen to her in a hospital. After I returned to school and then spent a number of years teaching undergraduate nurses about maternal–child nursing (and how to teach their patients), I started to formally study health education, and received my doctoral degree in that field from Columbia University. I learned all of the basics as well as the advanced information about how people learn, the best ways to teach them, and how to change behavior. I learned how to develop health education programs, and how to evaluate their effectiveness. I then went on to do research in the area, studying various health education interventions and how they worked for patients.

In my work with indigent, pregnant women in the Bronx, New York, I was always looking for appropriate patient education materials to share with them. Usually, I could find only handouts developed by pharmaceutical companies or formula companies—all heavily laden with product advertisements. Often it seemed to me that the material was written with an audience of college graduates in mind, because many of the pamphlets contained vocabulary was quite sophisticated. Rarely could I find anything for Spanish-speaking women. The cost of most of the commercially made health education pamphlets was prohibitive for my clinic (as I know it was for many others), so those materials were unavailable to me. Thus I began to develop patient education materials myself, and then evaluated how well they worked. As I became more well known through the articles I published in nursing journals, I was asked to speak about patient education at conferences around the country. Wherever I went across the United States to speak about patient education, nurses would tell me that they were desperate for quality health education materials for their patients, especially for materials translated into Spanish. Nurses also wanted handouts with minimal or no commercial endorsements in them. The idea for *Perinatal Patient Education* was born during that time.

Basically, this book is in two parts. Part I is designed to help nurses learn the basics of effective patient education. I've specifically designed Part I to be of use to working nurses. I didn't want it to be a textbook gathering dust on a shelf. I know that when you're working in the clinical area, the last thing you need is another textbook with pages and pages of words printed in small type. When you're on the job, you need information that is easy to

How To Use The Handouts In This Book

1. Don't tear the handouts out of the book! We have planned the binding of this book with plenty of room on the edges, so you can use a photocopier to copy the handouts. If you leave the handouts in the book, then you will always have the originals, and can never lose them!

2. Copy the handouts onto colored copy paper so they'll look interesting for the patients to read.

3. Although the handouts are grouped for convenience according to "Prenatal Health Education," "Intrapartum Care," "Postpartum Care," and "Interconceptional Care," in reality any of the handouts can be useful throughout or between pregnancies. Be sure to examine all of the handouts, no matter which area you work in. You might find, for instance, that handouts grouped in "Intrapartum Care" are appropriate to give to women in the third trimester of pregnancy.

4. Give the handouts to your patients. You can choose to give them out separately when the topic comes up in their care, or you can make folders for your patients, putting the appropriate handouts in each folder in advance, then giving the folders to your patients at the appropriate time. Perhaps intrapartum nurses will want to make folders containing all of the handouts on intrapartum topics to give to their patients who come in early labor. Prenatal nurses might want to develop folders for each trimester of pregnancy, placing the appropriate handouts in the folders. Mother–baby nurses might develop folders for their postpartum teaching duties, so the patients have something to take home.

5. If you are using the CD-ROM that comes with this book, you might want to have that CD available on your unit at all times, then you won't have to keep making copies of handouts. Whenever you need a handout about a particular topic, you can simply go to the computer, put in the CD-ROM, and print out the topic you need.

6. Whenever possible, ask the patients to read the material while you are still with them.

7. Review the material with your patients.

8. Ask the patients if they understand the material.

9. Ask the patients to restate what they've learned.

10. Ask the patients if they have any other questions.

access and easy to read. That's why Part I, with its important information that can help you be a better patient educator, is arranged with many bulleted lists and large headings. Hopefully that will make it easier to use and more accessible for in-service education programs for nurses.

Part II is the resource I always wanted when my primary job was teaching patients. It contains perinatal health education handouts for patients on most topics of interest to pregnant women—English on one side and Spanish on the other. Each handout is one side of one page and can be customized with the name of your institution, clinic, or office. The material has been written to help the average woman learn the most important things about a particular topic. Research has shown that we shouldn't give a huge amount of information to women about a topic and expect them to read or

remember it, so these handouts are "just the facts." They are designed for prenatal, intrapartum, and postpartum nurses to use as described in the box above.

Asking the patient to restate what she understood is essential. Each handout has a readability level between the 6th and 8th grades (with the readability grade level printed at the bottom of each handout).

The Spanish has been meticulously translated by expert nurse practitioners, Yovan Gonzalez and Zaida Betancourt Garcia. They read the English handouts, then wrote the Spanish handouts in "general Spanish." They asked people from many different Hispanic backgrounds to read the materials, because general Spanish can be understood by most Spanish-speaking adults, no matter which Spanish-speaking country they come from. We understand fully that some Latinas will say that a certain phrase might be written differently in their dialect, but because it is not possible to translate for each separate country of origin, we have correctly chosen "general Spanish." This should more than meet the needs of women for whom Spanish is their first language, or women who read better in Spanish than in English.

We know this book will fill two important needs that perinatal nurses have expressed: easy-to-use information about how patient education is best offered, and high-quality patient education materials for their patients that explain the most important facts about pregnancy. The Spanish translations have been painstakingly carried out, and will be invaluable for all nurses who work with those populations. I hope that someday I will be able to provide translations of these materials in other languages as well, and that I will be able to offer handouts for other areas of women's health besides pregnancy.

In thinking about why I wanted to write this book for nurses, it seems to me that Florence Nightingale said it best, way back in 1869, when nursing was the exclusive domain of women: "The following rules are by no means intended as a rule of thought by which nurses can teach themselves to nurse. . . they are meant simply to give hints for thought to women who have personal charge of the health of others. I do not pretend to teach her how. . . I ask her to teach herself, and for this purpose I venture to give her some hints."(Nightingale, 1869, p. 1)

Please let me know how you use this book and which parts are particularly beneficial. My aim has been to write a book that would be the most helpful to working nurses, and I hope I've accomplished that. I welcome your comments.

Margaret Comerford Freda, EdD, RN, CHES, FAAN
margaretfreda@yahoo.com

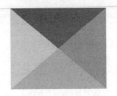

Acknowledgments

My interest in helping women learn more about their bodies and their pregnancies began when I was a labor and delivery nurse, and it was nurtured by many colleagues through the years. These people deserve special thanks for the parts they have played in my career, or in this book.

Karla Damus, PhD, RN, has been my mentor and friend for several decades. Her mentorship has meant the world to me. No colleague has taught me more, or given me more professional opportunities. Words cannot adequately express what Karla has done for me; my career would have been entirely different without her. Nancy DeVore, MS, CNM, asked me to help her educate indigent women in the Bronx, and thus was born my career in developing health education materials. Our collaboration over the years has been both professionally and personally gratifying. I have learned much from her, and thank her for her years of friendship. Irwin R. Merkatz, MD, has been my champion for the past 20 years, and has always encouraged me to accomplish whatever I desired. He is the chairman most people only dream of working for. I can never thank him enough for all he has done for me, and for all the doors he has opened for me.

Kathleen Rice Simpson, PhD, RN, FAAN, and Mary Brucker, DNS, CNM, read and critiqued every word of this book. They ensured that I kept regional practice issues in mind, helped to strengthen the cultural competence of the content, corrected my mistakes, and noticed all of my omissions. They were completely dedicated to making sure that the handouts were as good as they could possibly be. I am indebted to them in multiple ways, and I thank them for their time, their knowledge, their forthrightness, and their wonderful friendship.

Katie Capitulo, DNSc(c), RN, and Jane Corrarino, MSN, RN, read Part I of this book and provided many helpful comments, all of which made the content stronger. They are valued experts in patient education, and freely gave of their expertise. They have made this book far better than it would have been without their help.

Yovan Gonzalez, RN, and Zaida Betancourt Garcia, RN, were the expert nurses who provided the Spanish translations. They labored long and hard to make the Spanish content appropriate. I so appreciate all their efforts for this project. Muchas gracias.

Jennifer Brogan and Susan Rainey of Lippincott Williams & Wilkins have been enthusiastic about this book ever since I proposed it. Their dedicated editing and guidance have been appreciated daily as I wrote and rewrote. They are the miracle workers who even convinced a publishing company to publish a book that purposely allows its readers to copy parts of it and hand them out to others! I thank them for all they have done, and all they continue to do.

I thank my daughters Alyse and Carrie for being, in a word, perfect. No matter what I have done over the years, they have been there cheering for me. Another graduation from yet another school? No problem, they'd be there. In the recent past, even when their lives were disrupted, they showed the grace and spirit of the extraordinarily loving and kind young women they are. When times have called for it, they have been my solace. They teach me every day what it means to be empathetic and what life is truly about. I am the luckiest of women. What could be better?

Last, but first, is my husband of 35 years, John. His truthfulness, his integrity, his generosity, and his strength continue to amaze me. No matter the challenge, he has met it. No matter the circumstances, he is the voice of reason. He inhabits his multiple roles as husband, father, and grandfather with zest and unending love. None are his equal. Te amo, stranger on the shore.

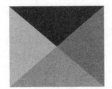

Contents

part II
Patient Education Handouts

Perinatal Patient Education

part I

Principles
of Education

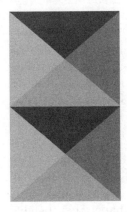

chapter 1

Basic Principles and Goals of Patient Education

Nurses have always considered health education an integral component of nursing care (Mason, 2001; Saarmann, Daugherty, & Riegel, 2000). Although we are often overworked and rushed in our daily lives as nurses, we never feel that we have completed our mission as nurses unless we have taught our patients what they need to know about their health, their condition, or their illness. We are unique among health care providers in this respect. Because we truly care about teaching our patients, it is frustrating for us when we don't have appropriate materials with which to teach them. We know that our patients learn better and remember more when they are given take-home materials, but finding and then paying for those materials can be a burden.

Not only must we find appropriate materials for teaching, but also we must consider how we are delivering information and education to our patients. Teaching and communication methods can influence how well the women will understand their condition as well as influence their ability to make informed choices (Blankson, Goldenberg, & Keith, 1994; Healton, Taylor, Burr, Dumois, Lowenstein, & Kaye, 1996; Redman, 1997). Where is the balance between imparting information and frightening the women we serve?

The Expert Panel on the Content of Prenatal Care of the United States Public Health Service has said that every encounter with a pregnant woman should be an educational encounter (U.S. Public Health Service, 1989). Prenatal care should not be just a series of physical examinations and laboratory tests, but an interactive experience that includes education about all aspects of pregnancy. Many times, it is not only the routine information that needs to be imparted, but also teaching about high-risk conditions, such as gestational diabetes or pregnancy-induced hypertension. Complicated screening tests, such as the Triple Screen or Maternal Serum Alpha Fetoprotein (MSAFP) testing, must also be explained to obtain informed consent (Freda, DeVore, Valentine-Adams, Bombard, & Merkatz, 1998).

Teaching and Learning Don't Go Hand in Hand

When we teach our patients, we assume they have learned what we taught. But have they? Do we know how much of our explanations they actually hear? When the woman leaves the office, clinic, hospital or birthing center, how much does she remember about what you taught? After your teaching, does she know enough to make the choices about lifestyle changes needed to improve her chance of an optimal outcome? What are her misconceptions, and will those misconceptions prevent her from carrying out the plan of care? Will her family assist or hinder her? Will her cultural beliefs interfere with or enhance the plan of care? Is she capable of performing the tasks you ask of her? All of these questions are essential to understanding the appropriate provision of health education for your patients. This book should help you to know the answers to these questions whenever you teach your patients.

Goal of Patient Education

It is important that we understand why we are engaged in educating our patients. It is tempting to believe that we educate our patients to help them follow our instructions more fully, but that is not the case.

BOX 1-1

The goal of patient education is to assist patients in the improvement of their own health.

This goal is accomplished by educating them about their bodies, their health, their condition, their illness, and their options, thus helping them to make informed decisions concerning treatment (Glanville, 2000). We can teach and we can help them to learn, but they will make the ultimate choice of behaviors and actions. That's why the terms "compliance"and "noncompliance" are rarely used these days. Once we have done our best to teach women properly, they then have the choice of whether or not to act on our teaching. Once we are sure that they did indeed understand what we taught them, they choose their own path. They are not "noncompliant" if they disagree with what we have urged them to do. Health care delivery is a partnership between patient and provider. If patients choose to disregard our teaching, that is their choice. Our job is to give our patients the knowledge to help them make their own decisions. If we know we've done our best to teach them properly, then we can accept the choices they make concerning their own health and their pregnancy.

Motivation to Learn

Motivation to learn is an essential component of the teaching process. No matter how good our teaching, if our patients are not motivated to learn, they can choose not to listen or to listen selectively. For instance, we might suggest to our patients that they stop smoking, lose weight, or start exercising. However, whether our patients are ready to learn that lesson and act on it are the keys to whether their behavior will change. Those of us who work with perinatal patients are particularly fortunate because pregnancy has been called the "teachable moment," that special time when most, but not all, women are interested in learning and are willing to modify behaviors that could affect pregnancy outcome (Calabro, Taylor, & Kapadia, 1996; Corrarino, Freda, & Barbara, 1995; Freda, Abruzzo, Davini, DeVore, Damus, & Merkatz, 1994).

Motivation to learn cannot be assumed, however, even during pregnancy. Although most women are motivated by the hope of an optimal pregnancy outcome, there are other women who may not be willing or able to change their behaviors. Women addicted to street drugs in pregnancy, for instance, may avoid prenatal care and the educational interventions inherent therein, fearing detection by the criminal justice system or fearing a reprimand by nurses or doctors. However, these women, too, can be motivated. Kearney and colleagues found that women who are actively using illicit drugs will be more likely to attend prenatal care when they believe that the prenatal care is an asset to improve fetal outcome and when they are not threatened with loss of child custody (Kearney, Murphy, Irwin, & Rosenbaum, 1995; Kearney, 1997). By understanding the motivation for learning, even in special situations such as this, nurses can be better able to structure educational experiences that emphasize motivating factors.

Some General Guidelines for the Provision of Effective Patient Education

There are three guidelines that are most helpful in conducting patient education. They are Simplicity, Reinforcement, and Sensitivity.

Simplicity

- **Assess** what the woman knows about the topic before you begin teaching.
- **Don't overteach.** When planning a teaching session, take some time before you begin to think about the **three or four most important things** for the woman to know about that topic. Then, teach only those topics. This is a difficult thing for most nurses to do. You want to be thorough, but in reality it is not possible or feasible to teach the woman everything you know about a topic. Trying to do so will only confuse her, so don't overteach.

- **Teach the simple concepts** about the diagnosis and treatment before you teach the complex ones.
- **Communicate at the woman's level of understanding.** Don't use medical terminology unless the woman is a perinatal health care professional.
- **Be aware of literacy issues** and the educational level of the woman. Check the readability of the materials you hand out—are they written at too high a level? (See Readability in Chapter 4.)
- **Be aware of the words you use.** To the general public, for instance, the word "positive" is a good thing, whereas in health care it often is not (think about "HIV positive"). There are many examples of poor word choice during teaching. One example is the term "intrauterine growth retardation," which can be easily misunderstood by women. For this term, we should make every effort to use the word "restriction," not "retardation," because women hear "retardation" and have every right to assume that we mean mental retardation, because that is the common use of the word (Freda, 1995).
- **Be concrete.** Tell the woman exactly what you mean and exactly what she needs to do. If you want the woman to come back to the hospital or birthing center when her contractions are 5 minutes apart, lasting 1 minute each for the past hour, then say so! Don't say "Call when you are in active labor."

Reinforcement

- **Present the most important information first, and then present it again last.** Take the time to decide what single piece of information is the most important take-home message, and be sure you repeat it.
- **Always reinforce what you've taught with written materials.** Our patients typically forget 50% of everything we say to them, so written materials they can take home can enhance learning by giving them additional opportunities to read the message we want to send.
- **Use visual aids if possible.**
- **Ask the woman to restate what you have taught.** How often do we tell a patient something, and then find out that she misinterpreted what we said? Listen carefully when she restates the teaching. Listen for myths and misinformation, and correct them.

Sensitivity

- **Be aware of the woman's culture.** If her culture is different than your own, do everything you can to learn more about her culture, because culture can be a major factor in learning. (See Cultural Competence in Chapter 5 for more information.)
- **Involve the family** in the education if possible. That way, even if the woman forgets some of what was taught, the family member might remember it. Family can also be helpful in assisting the woman toward behavior change. Remember that ``family'' is defined by the woman herself.
- **Be alert for emotional cues.** Women who are crying or distracted cannot listen or learn. If the woman is too upset about her new diagnosis or about the bad news about her pregnancy, wait until she is calm before initiating the teaching session.

In the next chapter, you'll learn all about the best methods for helping adults to learn.

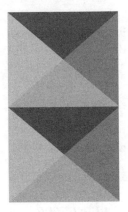

chapter 2

Adult Learning Principles

Those of us who work in the perinatal area usually work with adults or adolescents. Adults learn differently than children, and principles developed for classroom teaching of children are not necessarily useful in the teaching of adults. Adult learning principles, developed by Knowles (1980), tell us that adults learn best under certain circumstances. These adult learning principles are important for all patient educators to understand if we hope to assist women to learn as much as is needed during a pregnancy.

Adult Learning Principles (Knowles, 1980)

Principle #1. Adults learn best in response to a perceived need.

Principle #2. Teaching of adults should progress from what they already know to the unknown.

Principle #3. Teaching of adults should progress from simple concepts to the more complex concepts.

Principle #4. Adults learn best using active participation rather than passive listening.

Principle #5. Adults require opportunities to practice new skills with the teacher.

Principle #6. It's important to reinforce the desired behavior to enhance learning.

Principle #7. Immediate feedback and correction of misconceptions increase learning.

How to Use Adult Learning Principles for Patient Education

These principles can guide us in planning teaching for pregnant women. Every nurse who wants to be a good patient educator can use these principles every day. Let's see how that can be done.

EXAMPLE: Using the Adult Learning Principles for Teaching a Pregnant Woman About the Symptoms of Preterm Labor

■ **Principle #1**

Because *adults learn best in response to a perceived need*, engage the woman in a discussion of the problem of preterm birth and her particular risk. The severe health implications of preterm birth for the preterm infant can be emphasized so that the woman understands that although she might not perceive herself to be at risk, risk does exist in her pregnancy, as it does in all pregnancies.

■ **Principle #2**

She should then be *assessed for what she already knows* about the topic, so you can *progress from what she knows to the unknown*. Ask her what she knows about preterm birth. Ask her if she ever had a preterm birth or if she knows anyone who has. What have people told her about preterm birth? There are often myths in families or in cultures that need to be addressed. Myths are formidable and are often internalized at an early age and understood to be the absolute truth (Koff & Rierdan, 1995; Levinson, 1995; Myhre, 1996). Because the woman considers these myths to be true, it is not likely that she will bring them up in the context of a patient education session unless the nurse specifically asks what the woman knows about this topic. Myths must be addressed in a direct and forthright manner. When teaching about preterm birth, for example, the provider should ask what the woman's family or friends have told her about babies being born too early. In my 17 years of teaching women about this topic, for instance, I have found that there is a *predominating myth among some cultural groups that a baby born at 7 months' gestation is healthier than a baby born at 8 months' gestation*. This myth, which we as nurses recognize as clearly false as well as dangerous, is passed from grandmother to mother to daughter, making it difficult to convince women who have preterm labor symptoms at 28 weeks' gestation that they should seek care to avoid delivery at that time. Unless we ask women to tell us what they've been told by others about a topic, we might never have a chance to correct their misinformation.

▌ Principle #3

When teaching the woman about preterm birth, *the lesson should proceed from the simple concept* of why babies need at least 37 weeks of gestation to have the best chance of being born healthy, to the more detailed teaching of the subtle symptoms of preterm labor, to the particular instructions for what to do if symptoms develop, and then to the more complex concepts of how to access care if symptoms develop and what treatments might be offered. Teaching women about the use of antenatal glucocorticoids, for instance, includes informing the women that the drugs must be given to the mother about 24 hours before they become effective for maturing the baby's lungs. This is a complex concept. Unless the woman first understands about the dangers of respiratory distress syndrome, the concept of accessing care early enough to be given medication to delay its effects can be lost. When teaching about this topic, it is also important to impress upon women that preterm birth is still dangerous, despite the availability of antenatal corticosteroids to help mature fetal lungs. Some women believe that a premature labor is a shorter labor with an easier birth process. They need to understand that the availability of antenatal corticosteroids is important as an emergency measure, but these drugs do not alleviate all the other health problems faced by preterm infants.

▌ Principle #4

Because *active participation, rather than passive listening, promotes learning* in adults, each concept in the teaching should be addressed in a discussion format with the woman, not in a lecture format. Ask the woman meaningful questions throughout the lesson to encourage active participation. ***"Do you understand?" is not a meaningful question,*** because it requires only a "yes" or "no" answer. The woman who is shy, the woman whose first language is not English, or the woman who is embarrassed to admit she really doesn't understand what she has been taught, might answer "yes" to avoid feeling stupid. **Ask open-ended questions that require the woman to restate the portion of the lesson that just occurred ("Now, please tell me what you remember about the symptoms of preterm labor").**

▌ Principle #5

Because preterm labor teaching requires that the woman be taught to palpate for contractions, be sure that the woman *practices that skill during the lesson* so she feels confident that she truly understands where to place her fingers and what she is feeling.

▌ Principle #6

Reinforcement of the behavior can be encouraged by asking the woman to tell you just how she would go about dealing with preterm symptoms in specific conditions (what if the symptoms develop when she's at work, for example, or when she's in the park with her other children). Invent a scenario in which the woman experiences symptoms and elicit her response about how she would handle that situation.

▌ Principle #7

Providing immediate feedback to the woman on how she handled the fictitious situation will help to correct any misconceptions she might have and will also reassure you that the teaching session has provided the woman with needed decision-making skills should the symptoms appear.

Now go on to the next chapter to discover how we as nurses can influence our patients to change their behaviors in reponse to our teaching.

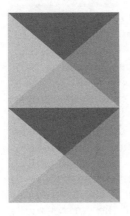

chapter 3

Behavior Change Principles

Models of Behavior Change

We know that knowledge alone does not change behavior. Most of us can look to our own lives and realize that just because we know, for example, that daily exercise is good for health, doesn't mean that we all exercise every day. Some of us smoke cigarettes, eat fast foods, skip breakfast, weigh too much, diet too much, or drive too fast. We know that those things aren't good for us, but we do them anyway. Our patients behave the same way. Even if we teach them the best ways to stay healthy during pregnancy, they still might not change the behaviors that need changing. The decision to change their behavior is ultimately theirs, but it is our duty to provide them with information so they can make informed choices. The question of how we can help them to make behavioral changes is all-important.

First, we should become familiar with the subject of behavior change and know how to influence it. We don't have to leave it up to chance to figure out how and why people change behaviors. Many learned scholars have studied this topic, and we can use the knowledge they've generated to help us help our patients. There are several models that help us to understand how and why people change their behavior (Bandura & Adams, 1982; Becker, 1974; Becker & Janz, 1985; Grimley, Prochaska, Velicer, & Prochaska, 1996; Janz & Becker, 1984; Prochaska, 1994). Why is it important to understand these models? Because they give us a window into a better understanding of human behavior. Models, also called theories and theoretical frameworks (remember them from your basic nursing program?), are simply ways of looking at the world or at a particular topic.

Let's look at a model outside of nursing as an example. Everyone is familiar with Freud and Freudian theory. If you are confronted with a child who is acting out destructively in school, for instance, and your theoretical framework (another way of saying your "model") is similar to that of Freud, you would believe that this child needs individual therapy to discover the root cause of his acting out (Freud, 1909). This child needs to learn why he acts as he does; only then can he change. If your model, however, is Murray Bowen, you would believe that all problems in life are related to basic problems within the family system (Bowen, 1978). If your model is Bowenian and you have a child who is acting out destructively, your best response is for the entire nuclear family to enter therapy together. The Bowen model tells us that the problem is not the child's alone; it exists within the family, and everyone in the family must acknowledge his or her part in it before it can be overcome.

Likewise, if you want to know why people react in certain ways to health problems, you can look at various models of health behavior change. The following models of behavior change are simply three different ways of looking at how people change. You can choose the one that makes the most sense to you and then work with that.

Health Belief Model

One of the most commonly cited models of behavior change is the Health Belief Model, which has been used for several decades and helps us to understand why patients take or do not take action to improve their health (Becker, 1974). Using the Health Belief Model, behavior change is theorized to be a balance of three things.

Behavior change depends on the patient's:

1. **perceived susceptibility** to the disease.
2. **perceived benefits** from performing the behavior asked of her.
3. **perceived barriers** to performing the behavior.

EXAMPLE: Gestational Diabetes From the Health Belief Model Framework

Let's look at gestational diabetes as an example of how you can use the Health Belief Model. We all know that gestational diabetes is a diagnosis in pregnancy that should ultimately result in behavior change. The woman has to accept her diagnosis, change her eating habits, and usually learn how to use a syringe, inject insulin, and administer it to herself properly. All of that is extremely difficult behavior change. How can the Health Belief Model account for how this behavior change occurs?

1. **"Perceived susceptibility":** The Health Belief Model tells us that a woman diagnosed with gestational diabetes has to believe that the disease is a reality. She has to ***believe that she is susceptible to this illness***. If she has no symptoms, for instance, she might not want to believe that there really is anything wrong with her. Your part as a nurse is therefore to stress objective findings, such as the laboratory reports and the ultrasound findings of a large-for-gestational-age baby. This can help to make the condition more real for the affected woman.
2. **"Perceived benefits":** The treatment regimen for gestational diabetes is rigorous. The woman has to understand ***what benefits she will gain from learning*** to test her blood sugar, use a syringe, and inject insulin several times a day. She needs to be taught about why control of gestational diabetes can lead to a healthier fetus.
3. **"Perceived barriers":** The woman then has to balance the benefits of treatment with the ***bar-riers in her life that could interfere with compliance with the treatment plan***. There might be multiple barriers. For instance, does she have medical insurance that will pay for the insulin and syringes, or does she have to pay for supplies herself? Lack of money can be a major barrier. Does she lack confidence in her ability to learn how to handle syringes, a task that is frightening to most adults and that might be equated with the illicit drug culture for others? Fear is another strong barrier to treatment. Does she have a support system at home to help her purchase the correct foods and help her manage this illness? Lack of a support system can be the barrier that causes her to miss her follow-up appointments or to stray from her diabetic diet.

Only when the perceived benefits outweigh the perceived barriers in her own mind will she learn the tasks and perform the behavior.

It is your job as the nurse who teaches this woman to help her see that the benefits outweigh the barriers. You cannot do this job well until you have assessed all the barriers to behavior change in this individual woman's life.

Many researchers have studied behavior change using the Health Belief Model and have found that **perceived barriers are the most powerful part of the model** (Janz & Becker, 1984). What does that mean for us, the patient educators? It means that, despite all we might teach a woman about the importance of injecting herself with insulin to treat gestational diabetes, if she has too many "perceived barriers," she might not be able to comply with the care you suggest. Knowing this about the Health Belief Model, you can plan your teaching to include talking at length with the woman about the barriers to treatment that she perceives. If you can help her to overcome the barriers, you can help her to change her behavior. This model has been studied with hypertension, asthma, obesity, medication taking, regimen adherence, cancer screening, and appointment keeping, among other health issues (Becker & Janz, 1985; Davis et al., 2001). It is a powerful way for us to understand behavior change and to help our patients attain goals of healthy behavior. See Box 3-1.

Transtheoretical Stages of Change

A newer model explaining why and how people change their behavior is the Transtheoretical Stages of Change Model, which assists the nurse to anticipate the woman's readiness for change

BOX 3-1
The Health Belief Model

The Health Belief Model helps us to understand that our patients will respond if they perceive they are susceptible, if they understand that the risk is serious, if they learn that they will benefit from the treatment, and especially if the barriers to adherence can be overcome.

(Grimley et al., 1996; Prochaska, 1994). If you use this model, you see change as a series of stages. Before a patient can move to the next level, she must have accomplished the previous stage. The stages of change are as follows:

1. Precontemplation
2. Contemplation
3. Preparation
4. Action
5. Maintenance

EXAMPLE: Smoking Cessation From the Transtheoretical Stages of Change Model

Let's see just how this model would work when a nurse wants to do some teaching. **The first step in using this model is assessing the apparent stage of the woman in question.**

If a woman is in the *Precontemplative* stage, for instance, it is virtually impossible to ask her to move directly to an "Action" stage. For example, a pregnant woman who has never thought about giving up her usual high-fat, fast-food daily lunch during pregnancy (she has not *contemplated* any change and doesn't even see its necessity) will more than likely not respond to you saying, "You need to stop eating a Big Mac, french fries, and a milkshake every day for lunch."

The best way to discover which stage a woman is in is to ask some questions. If you want to help a woman stop smoking but you don't know if she is ready to quit, for instance, you might ask "Have you ever thought about stopping smoking?" If the woman answers "No," and says that smoking helps to calm her down, then it won't do any good to give her the address of a smoking cessation clinic. For a woman in this precontemplation stage, time must be spent educating her about the dangers of cigarette smoke to her and to the fetus. That teaching can move

the woman from a precontemplation to the next stage (Todd, La Sala, & Neil-Urban, 2001).

If the woman's answer to your question about smoking is "Yes, I've thought about it, but I just can't seem to do it," then the woman has moved past the precontemplation stage toward the *Contemplation* stage. Many pregnant women are in the contemplation stage concerning health issues such as smoking, because they want to have a healthy pregnancy and healthy baby. For a woman in the contemplation stage, additional information about the danger of cigarettes can be helpful, but you really want to focus on how smoking cessation is accomplished and where the smoking cessation clinics are located.

Some women are in the *Preparation* stage, meaning they've decided to stop smoking, but just haven't actually done it yet. For a woman like this, who has already decided to stop smoking, it is not necessary to spend time and effort teaching about the dangers of cigarettes. Give the woman the telephone numbers of smoking cessation clinics or programs. Help her to make an appointment to start the program, and ask her to set a deadline for when this will be done. Congratulate her on her decision to stop smoking, and talk to her about how she's going to avoid her usual triggers to smoking.

A woman in the *Action* stage is already working on smoking cessation, and your efforts should be directed toward support and encouragement at each visit. In a situation such as this, it's a good idea to praise her for the action she has taken and even ensure that other health care providers tell her what a great job she has done in stopping smoking. Every time you see her in the office or clinic, praise her!

In the *Maintenance* stage, when the woman has stopped smoking and is trying to stay cigarette free, you should provide active support and encouragement, because everyone knows it is easy to slip back into smoking when anxiety or upset occurs. Help the woman to use the skills she used in her smoking cessation program when she feels the need to smoke. If she relapses and starts to smoke again, talk to her about the challenges of smoking cessation and assure her that she can quit again. If relapse occurs, do not become judgmental. Assess what stage the woman is currently in, and begin the process of helping her to quit again. See Box 3-2.

Self-Efficacy Theory

Self-efficacy theory (Bandura & Adams, 1982) is a third theory of behavior change, useful to the

BOX 3-2
The Transtheoretical Stages of Change

The Transtheoretical Stages of Change Model tells us that if we find out what stage of change a person is in before we start our patient education, we will have a better chance of helping him or her to accomplish the behavior change.

BOX 3-3
Self-Efficacy Theory

Self-Efficacy Theory tells us that partitioning the behavior change into manageable parts can help the person to believe that behavior change is possible.

nurse who provides patient education. *This theory states that a patient must first believe that change is possible before change can occur.* A person with high self-efficacy will be more likely to change a behavior. This theory of behavior change fits very well when your patient might feel like a victim, either of an illness or in a relationship.

EXAMPLE: Violence and Abuse From the Self-Efficacy Model

Perhaps your patient is involved in a violent relationship. You know this, and decide to discuss domestic violence with her. When you talk to her, it is clear to you that the woman does not believe it is even possible for her to live a life free of violence. She cannot imagine any way that she can get away from her abuser. In this instance, helping the woman to increase her self-efficacy is the appropriate course of action to help activate behavior change. How do you help the woman increase her self-efficacy? You help her to see that behavior change is, indeed, possible, even when she thinks it isn't. You can help her to believe this by partitioning the behavior change into smaller easier subtasks. Asking (or worse, telling) the woman with low self-efficacy to leave the abuser will not promote behavior change. Instead, your first step would be to ask her to just start thinking about what her life would be like if she felt

safe. This is the first subtask. You can talk to her about feeling safe and how good she would feel if she and her children could feel safe again. She just has to consider it.

At her next visit, you can ask what she's been thinking about. If she has thought about even the possibility of feeling safe again, you can help her to move to a second subtask: beginning a "safety plan." You can sit with her privately and explain the concept of a safety plan. Discuss all the possibilities for how she could plan for the day when she and her children would be safe. A safety plan includes plans to hide money, to make extra keys for the car and hide them, for emergency shelter with a friend or relative who would take her in, and to keep a bag packed and hidden for herself and her children that contains her marriage license, her bank account numbers, her insurance policy numbers, rent and utility receipts, important phone numbers, and the social security numbers of her husband, her children, and herself (McFarlane & Gondolf, 1998).

By discussing her thoughts about escape plans and adding your input, you are recognizing and rewarding this woman for taking some first small steps toward eventual success. Each succeeding visit will elicit one more small step until the small behavioral changes become additive. Thus self-efficacy grows, the escape plan is completed, and the woman is able to contemplate acting on it. See Box 3-3.

The next chapter discusses the important issues of literacy and readability as they relate to patient education.

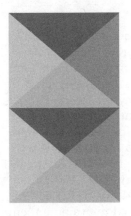

chapter 4

Readability/Literacy/ Low Literacy

Readability/Literacy

We know from health education research that written information that accompanies oral teaching enhances the patient's understanding of what was taught. Therefore, every patient education session should end with the provision of appropriate written information for the woman to take home (Arthur, 1995; Doak, Doak, & Root, 1996; Glanville, 2000). I must emphasize, however, that it is *essential* that the content of the written information be appropriate for the woman. A patient education booklet or information sheet that contains huge amounts of technical information or that is written at an inappropriate reading level will not educate patients (Estey, Musseau, & Keenan, 1994). It is therefore incumbent upon us as nurses to ensure that the materials we provide for our patients are at the appropriate reading level, and that we use strategies known to make educational materials readable and interesting to patients.

How Can We Tell How Well Our Patients Read?

Finding out how well a person reads is not easy. Most nurses, if they want to know how well their patients can read, would look at the medical record to find out the "last grade completed" and then assume that the person reads at that level. If, for instance, the person finished 12th grade, you might assume that she reads well. In fact, however, literacy does not equate with grade level; as a matter of fact, most patients' reading levels are 3 to 5 years below their completed grade level

(Doak et al., 1996). Murphy, Chesson, Berman, Arnold, and Galloway (2001) have recently reported this for their population, which had a mean educational level of 12th grade. When Murphy and colleagues tested their population's actual reading grade level, however, it was at the 7th to 8th grade. Not only are grade level and reading level poorly correlated, but you might be surprised to learn that the average reading level of citizens of the United States is at the 8th-grade level. Even more surprising to most people is that about 1 in 5 people in the United States read at the 5th-grade level or below (Doak et al., 1996). Most newspapers in the United States are written at the 9th to 12th grade reading levels; that means that about 20% of Americans cannot read and understand them!

If you are concerned about your particular population's reading ability, there are scientific ways that you can discover how well your patient population reads. For most working nurses, the use of these methods is far too time consuming, but if you are interested in doing research in the area of patient education, you might want to test your patient population's reading ability. Some tests used for this purpose are the Wide Range Achievement Test (WRAT) and the Rapid Estimate of Adult Literacy in Medicine (REALM) (Doak et al., 1996). It is beyond the purpose of this book to prepare you to administer such tests. Be aware, however, that using these tests and all others that examine a person's ability to read can make patients feel uncomfortable and worried that they will not be considered smart if they cannot read. You can assure them, though, that reading ability is not correlated with IQ (Redman, 1997). Not being able to read well usually means that a person just wasn't taught to read, or hasn't practiced reading, or perhaps has an undiagnosed learning disability. If you choose to use reading ability tests, you must prepare the patients well and be sure to be empathetic about their results.

What Readability Level Is Appropriate for Health Education Materials?

Readability is the ease with which a person can read and understand the written word. Health education experts agree that materials developed for the general public should be written between the 6th- and 8th-grade reading levels to ensure that the largest number of people can read them and follow their directions (Doak et al., 1996; Redman, 1997). Health education materials, however, must necessarily include some words not normally found in general materials ("hysterectomy," "alpha-fetoprotein," "amniotic fluid," "Kegel," "preeclampsia," etc.). These words alone could make the readability score higher, so it is even more important that all the other words in the handout be made as simple to read as possible. In this book, all of the health education materials will be labeled with their reading level according to the Flesch-Kincaid Reading Level formula. That formula was calculated with the Readability Calculator, a software program manufactured by Micro Power and Light (Dallas, TX). All of the handouts in this book are between the 6th- and 8th-grade readability levels.

Don't Most Patient Education Materials Take Readability Into Account?

I wish the answer to that question was "yes," but unfortunately it is not. It has been shown that most health education materials are written at readability levels that are far above the average reader's reading level, and are therefore incomprehensible to a significant number of patients (Albright, deGuzman, Acebo, Paiva, Faulkner, & Swanson, 1996; Arthur, 1995; Ayello, 1993; Beaver & Luker, 1997; Brownsen, 1998; Doak et al., 1996; Dowe, Lawrence, Carlson, Kerseling, 1997; Estey et al., 1994; Lindau, Tomori, McCarville, & Bennett, 2001; Maynard, 1999). This has been studied in many different settings, with many different types of health education materials, and unfortunately the results are always the same. Davis and colleagues (1994) found that 80% of materials produced by the

American Academy of Pediatrics, the Centers for Disease Control, and pharmaceutical companies were written at the 10th-grade reading level. Analysis of consent forms from the National Cancer Institute found all to be at readability levels of grades 12–17 (Meade & Howser, 1992). Patient information booklets from the American College of Obstetricians and Gynecologists (ACOG) have been analyzed twice. In 1988 the materials were evaluated at grades 11 and higher (Zion & Aiman, 1989) and in 1998, readability of all 100 patient education pamphlets ranged from 7.0 to 9.3, depending on the formula used to evaluate them (Freda, Damus, & Merkatz, 1999).

What if Your Patients Are Well Educated? Won't They Be Insulted by Materials Written at the 6th- to 8th-Grade Level?

Many studies have shown that when patients receive written information they recall what they were taught more fully (Meade, Byrd, & Lee, 1989). ***We also know that materials written at a lower readability level are more effective, no matter what the reading ability of the population*** (Calabro, Taylor, & Kapadia, 1996; Meade et al., 1989). Even if the population we serve is well educated, the simple language used in health education materials developed at the 6th to 8th-grade reading level has been shown to be better understood and recalled than materials developed at higher reading levels (Davis et al., 1994). All of us who provide patient education should be aware of the issue of readability and should not be using patient education materials that are written at much higher than the 6th to 8th-grade level, so that the majority of women can comprehend them (Estey et al., 1994).

How Can We Test the Readability of the Materials We Use for Patients?

Readability is tested with mathematical formulas. But don't worry—you don't have to memorize any mathematical formulas to do this. Testing the readability of the materials you use for your patients is really quite easy, as you will see in this chapter. Most often, readability formulas measure combinations of frequency of multisyllabic words and sentence length. There are many different formulas used for testing the readability of written materials; certain formulas are more appropriate for specific audiences, such as children, textbook readers, or adults. Although different formulas produce slightly different results, Meade and Smith (1991) have shown that results correlate highly with each other. For those of you who want to do research in this area, there are computer programs available that calculate the readability of patient educational materials according to several standardized formulas, such as Fog, Flesch-Kincaid, Fry, and SMOG (Redman, 1997). The Readability Calculator from Micro Power and Light is the software program I routinely use when evaluating readability.

There are several readability formulas that are most commonly used to evaluate health education materials. The most commonly used formulas, and what they do, are listed in Box 4-1.

Which Readability Formula Should You Use?

There has been research that shows that all the formulas are accurate and are reasonably well correlated with each other (Meade & Smith, 1991). So what is the working nurse to do with this information? Most of you will just want to examine the materials you are currently using for their readability levels or check the readability levels of the health-education materials you develop for your own patients. How should you do it? I recommend you choose the easiest path. As a practicing nurse, you are busy with multiple essential jobs that you must complete, so examining the readability of the materials you give your patients should be done as easily as possible. Rather than learning any calculations or purchasing any readability programs, I suggest you check readability using one of the two most commonly used word-processing programs these days: Microsoft Word or Corel's WordPerfect. I bet you're using one of them at home or at work for word processing. Both of these programs can calculate the readability grade level of whatever you type. Both of them use the **Flesch-Kincaid Grade Level formula.** Instructions for checking the readability of patient-education materials are included in Box 4-2.

For any other word-processing programs or for different versions of the programs I have mentioned, read your manual and find out if they calculate readability by a specific readability formula. If you don't have a manual, use the "Help" portion of the program and type in "readability statistics." If the program provides this function, it will tell you how to use it. If not, perhaps you can upgrade to one of these programs or borrow a computer that has one of these programs loaded into it. If you care about this topic, as I assume you do because you're reading this book, it will be worth it.

What to Do If the Materials You Check Are Higher Than the 8th-Grade Readability Level

If you check the materials you are using and they are consistently far above the recommended 6th- to 8th-grade level, you might want to consider using different materials (such as the ones in this book!), or developing materials yourself. Chapter 7 describes how to develop health-education materials for patients.

BOX 4-1
Commonly Used Readability Formulas

The **Fog formula** counts numbers of sentences and numbers of long words, emphasizing the difficulty level of the words. It is useful for grades 4 through college (Redman, 1997).

The **Flesch Reading Ease Score** rates the text on a 100-point scale. The higher the score, the easier it is to understand the text. It is based on average sentence length and average number of syllables per word (Doak et al., 1996).

The **Flesch-Kincaid Grade Level** calculates readability based on the length of sentences and words. A score of 10.2 on this formula means, for instance, that a person needs 10.2 years of education to successfully read the text. It is useful for grades 5 through college and is used by the U.S. Department of Health and Human Services for their educational materials (London, 1999).

The **Fry formula** calculates the ratio of number of syllables for each 100 words to the number of sentences per 100 words. It is used commonly with health-related materials, and can determine readability for grades 1 through 17, but should not be used for text with fewer than 300 words (Doak et al., 1996; Redman, 1997).

The **SMOG** formula counts numbers of sentences as well as numbers of words with three or more syllables. It is useful for grades 5 through college and predicts the grade level within 1.5 grades (Redman, 1997). It is a commonly used formula and doesn't require a computer, because it can be calculated by hand. The formula for computing SMOG readability can be found in Doak et al. (1996).

BOX 4-2

Checking the Readability of Your Patient Education Materials

For WordPerfect 8: Type in the material you want to check. It's a good idea if you type in the entire handout you are giving your patient, but if you have a very long document, you don't need to type in the entire document. You can type two paragraphs from the beginning, then two from the middle, and then two from the end of the document. When you've finished typing, go to Tools, then Grammatik, then Options, then Analysis, and then Readability. The Flesch-Kincaid Grade Level Score will appear. The ideal document should be between 6th- and 8th-grade readability. If so, it's probably a document that is readable by many women.

For WordPerfect 9: Block the areas that you want to check. Go to Grammatik, then Options, then Analysis, and then Readability. The Flesch-Kincaid Grade Level Score will appear.

For Microsoft Word 97: Type in the document as explained above. Then go to Tools, Spell, Options, and Show Readability. Again, the Flesch-Kincaid Grade Level will appear.

For Microsoft Word 2000: Type in the document as explained above. Then go to Tools. Click Options, then click Spelling and Grammar. Check the box "Check Grammar with Spelling." Check the box "Show Readability Statistics," then "OK." Click "Spelling and Grammar" on the Standard toolbar. When Word 2000 finishes checking spelling and grammar, it will display the Flesch-Kincaid readability score.

Low Literacy

There are very few patient educational materials that are specifically designed for pregnant women with low-literacy skills. This is too bad, because 1 in 5 Americans is functionally illiterate

(Weiss & Coyne, 1997). If you work with a population of women who have low-literacy skills, you will probably have to develop materials for them yourself. Corrarino, Freda, & Barbara (1995) did just that in a public health prenatal clinic in New York. Their article in the *Journal of Perinatal Education* is a good resource for this purpose (Corrarino et al. 1995). One of the best books I have encountered on this topic is by Doak, Doak, & Root. (1996). Below are some of the techniques they suggest for developing materials for women with low literacy.

Low-Literacy Strategies (Doak, 1996)

- Use large print.
- Do not use all capital letters (THEY ARE MORE DIFFICULT TO READ).
- Use **bold type** to emphasize important facts.
- Use an easy-to-read font such as **Times Roman.**
- Use short sentences and words with few syllables.
- Use illustrations that suggest the message wherever possible.
- Use horizontal lists, not vertical ones.
- Use the active voice.
- Use cues such as <u>underlining</u>, circles, and color to help guide the eye.
- Leave much blank space on each page.
- Use a question-and-answer format for written information.
- Use no more than 7 items in lists.
- Avoid double negatives.

Most of these suggestions, although made for low-literacy populations, work very well for patient education materials for patients with literacy levels higher than the 5th grade. If you work with a population of women with particularly low literacy, you must be even more careful with the written materials you give them. If no low-literacy materials are available, you might want to use videotapes for teaching, which can effectively teach women with poor reading skills. **The next chapter discusses the vital areas of cultural competence and informed consent in patient education.**

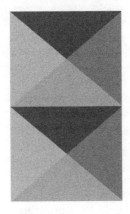

chapter 5

Cultural Competence/ Informed Consent

Cultural Competence in Patient Education

There is no doubt that culture influences the behavior of our patients and also influences the way they learn. We must, therefore, be cognizant of the cultural values and mores of the women we serve. When I was in nursing school we called this "cultural sensitivity," but the term used now is "cultural competence." This change has come about because it is perceived that when one is "sensitive" to another culture, the implication is that the nurse's culture is dominant (or even superior), and he or she must be "sensitive" to others. The newer concept of "cultural competence" suggests that no one culture is superior to another and that we must all be "competent" to work with people of many cultures (Freda, 1997; Sabogal, 1996). This change in terminology might seem like only an effort to be politically correct, but I think it makes sense, and I'm happy to adopt the term "cultural competence."

The Multicultural Milieu of the United States

As the American public becomes ever more ethnically diverse, nurses are faced with providing care and education to patients from cultures with which they may be completely unfamiliar. How, then, can patient education be accomplished in a culturally competent manner? First you will need to find out which cultures you are dealing with in your community and work toward learning more about those cultures. When you know, for instance, that there is a large Hmong population of pregnant women coming to your institution, clinic, or office, it is incumbent upon you to learn all you can about that culture so you can deliver care and patient education in a way the women find acceptable. Although some nurses might feel this is an additional burden placed upon them, actually developing an understanding of your patients' subjective culture, including some of the major beliefs, attitudes, roles, social norms, and values, can be an exciting and challenging addition to your nursing practice. It could even make your job easier!

How Can You Learn About Other Cultures?

Probably the best and most direct way is to ask questions. Talk to members of the cultural group you want to reach. Ask them what specific pregnancy beliefs or customs are inherent in their culture. Some cultures, for instance, frown upon any male provider caring for a woman. In some cultures there are strict rules about the placenta; it might be an obligation, for instance, to take the placenta home for ritual disposal (McCartney, 2000; Schneiderman, 1998). In some cultures, the concepts of "hot" and "cold" are essential during the postpartum period. Because the woman's body is believed to be in a "cold" state after giving birth, the woman needs to regain balance through the use of anything "hot," such as drinks, foods, or treatments. No cold foods can be eaten for the first month after giving birth (Davis, 2001).

The next step is to go to the nursing literature, in which there are numerous research articles about caring for women who come from cultures different than your own (Callister, Lauri, & Vehvilainen-Julkunen, 2000; Davis, 2001; Foss, 2001; Jones, Bond, Gardner, & Hernandez, 2002; Kridli, 2002; McCartney, 2000; York, Bhuttarowas, & Brown, 1999). There are also excellent books and monographs that detail the important cultural and health beliefs of multiple cultures. One such book in the form of a nursing module is produced by the March of Dimes Birth Defects Foundation (Moore & Moos, 2002).

After you have asked the women of the culture in your population, and after you have done some research in the literature about the culture of the patients you routinely provide care for, you will feel more comfortable that you understand some of that culture's basic beliefs about childbearing. Then you will be ready to help the women through patient education. It's entirely possible that your review of the literature might have pointed out that you need to re-consider the teaching methodologies you have relied on in the past. Researchers have found that the teaching methods one uses for one cultural group may not be effective with a different ethnic or cultural group. An instructive example is the use of "scare tactics," such as showing gruesome pictures of the end result if the patient doesn't listen to the health teaching. Health educators generally avoid using scare tactics, because we know from the literature that they are of little value in health education. Sabogal and colleagues, however, found that the use of scare tactics was actually very effective in working with a Vietnamese population, because their belief system includes a strong requirement to visualize the results of disease (Sabogal, 1996).

Sabogal's group has offered the following suggestions for how to develop a teaching program for a culture different than your own.

Developing a Teaching Program for a Culture Different Than Your Own (Sabogal, 1996)

- Be aware of your own assumptions, biases, and prejudices. Unless you know something directly from members of the cultural group or from scientific research done with that cultural group and published in a peer-reviewed journal, do not assume it to be true. Many generalizations we make about cultural groups are unfounded.
- Make every effort to understand the core cultural values of the group. For instance, Latinos

in Sabogal's study described a strong sense of family ("familismo"). This was used by the health care providers when they made sure that family was included in the education they provided, and the material taught included the implications of treatment options on the family. Another Latino cultural value identified was "fatalismo," a belief that little can be done to alter one's fate. This could significantly reduce the impact of health teaching if it is not addressed forthrightly as a part of the teaching. The Latino patients studied by Sabogal needed to be reminded repeatedly that treatment and cure were possible; stories from other affected Latino community members who had been treated successfully significantly improved the effectiveness of the teaching (Sabogal, 1996).

- If you are developing written materials for the target audience, ask a native speaker from that culture to read the material you developed in English and then to write that material in the appropriate language. Don't ask anyone to translate the material exactly from the English, because translations from English to another language are often impossible and often culturally irrelevant. There is a science to the translation process. You can read more about this in the article by Capitulo (Capitulo, Cornelio, & Lenz, 2001).
- Use testimonials of persons within the target audience as role models. If you or your colleagues are not of the target ethnic group, talk to patients or community members who could come to your session and vouch for your credibility. Testimonials build confidence, and an interested community member can be your best ally.

Informed Consent

One of the reasons nurses teach patients is to obtain informed consent for tests or procedures. Do you understand the legal ramifications of asking a patient to sign a consent form versus witnessing the signing of a consent form? There's a major difference between them.

- If you ask the patient to read and then sign the informed consent document, you are affirming that your patient understands enough about the ramifications of her diagnosis, procedure, or test to make an informed decision.

- ***In some institutions only the person who will actually be performing the procedure (such as the anesthesiologist or the physician or the midwife) can ask for the informed consent***. In those cases, **when you witness the informed consent, you are *only* affirming that it was indeed the patient who signed the document** (Cady, 2000).

In either case, however, you as a nurse and as the patient's advocate want to know that she understands the informed consent document. But does she really understand? I'm sorry to tell you that there is a large amount of literature that tells us that, when it comes to informed consent, our patients *rarely comprehend* or recall what we have taught them (Braddock, Fihn, Levinson, Jonsen, & Perlman, 1997; Earley, Blanco, Prien, & Willis, 1991; Faden, Chwalow, Orel-Crosby, Holtzman, Chase, & Leonard, 1985; Hekkenberg, Irish, Rotstein, Brown, & Gullane, 1997; Marteau, Johnston, Plenicar, Shaw, & Slack, 1988; Marteau, Kidd, Michie, Cook, Johnston, & Shaw, 1993). Despite this universally dismal outcome, very little has been done by the health care community to improve the teaching of patients from whom we request informed consent. Braddock and colleagues (1997), for instance, found that discussions in the primary care setting rarely assessed the patients' understanding of information presented by a physician. Hekkenberg et al. (1997) studied what patients understood after a teaching session about surgical complications and found that 50% of the surgical patients taught had flawed understanding of the complications from surgery. Other authors have suggested that the emotional distress associated with a medical decision makes comprehension difficult when informed consent is requested (Charles, Gafni, & Whelan, 1995; Klepatsky & Mahlmeister, 1997; Kuba, 1995; Pape, 1997; Sandelowski & Jones, 1996). In a study about whether pregnant women who were taught about maternal serum alpha-fetoprotein testing understood enough to fulfill the criteria for informed consent, it was found that although 80% of the women agreed to have the screening test, 38% of those women could not describe the purpose of the test, and 72% of the women thought that a negative test meant that their baby would be healthy in all respects (Freda, DeVore, Valentine-Adams, Bombard, & Merkatz, 1998). Similar misconceptions were also found in other studies of this subject (Faden et al., 1985; Marteau et al., 1993; Sikkink, 1990).

How Much of What We Teach Should Be Understood by Patients?

There is no agreement in the literature or in the legal system about what actually constitutes understanding of topics that require informed consent (Freda et al., 1998; Lurvey, Nager, & Johnson, 1996). Until further study of this issue is undertaken, therefore, nurses really have no standards to guide them for how much comprehension is acceptable. Is it okay if our patients can restate only 50% of what we taught them, or is 33% satisfactory? Do they need to understand 75% of the material? These questions have not yet been asked nor answered in the literature or in the law. Thus is it incumbent upon those of us who teach our patients and then request informed consent to evaluate what our patients really understand, and document our impressions. Andre (1993) has even suggested that providers should alter the way they think about informed consent, and that it should actually be considered an interactive process through which two people come to an understanding. Chervenak has recommended that informed consent be the vehicle through which an ongoing dialogue between pregnant women and their care providers can be fostered (Chervenak & McCullough, 1990). Searight (Searight & Barbarash, 1994) has recommended that informed consent be considered **strictly** a method for educating patients and that providers use the following set of five questions to evaluate patients' learning every time a new treatment, test, or procedure is suggested.

1. What do you call your condition?
2. Which treatment is being recommended?
3. What is the treatment supposed to do for you?
4. Are there risks associated with the treatment?
5. What alternatives are there to the treatment?

Because the goal of patient education is to assist the woman to understand enough about her condition to be able to make informed choices about treatment, and because the research shows that patients generally do not understand the complicated issues we teach them, it seems that changes should be made in the way we request informed consent. Searight's suggestion to use an interactive dialogue between provider and patient during which the patient is asked to restate the education given, describing the test or treatment and its ramifications, seems appropriate and long overdue. Unfortunately, the cost of such interactive processes involving dialogues between patients and nurses through which evaluation of patient learning can be assessed may not be possible in today's health care environment in which cost cutting seems rampant. Nurses need to work toward devising more effective ways to permit patients to have an educated voice in their own health care; one way of doing this is for nurses to become more knowledgeable themselves about how best to educate their patients.

Now go to the next chapter, which describes how patient education is best delivered.

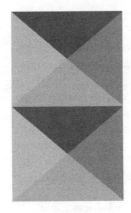

chapter 6

Methods of Providing Patient Education

Joint Commission on the Accreditation of Healthcare Organizations' Goals

The Joint Commission on the Accreditation of Healthcare Organizations (JCAHO) first added patient and family education outcomes as a high priority and a focus survey area in 1993 (Rankin & Stallings, 2001). This leadership on the part of JCAHO validates nursing's long-standing position that patient education is an integral component of comprehensive care. Because of these initiatives, patient and family education is now seen as essential in promoting healthy behaviors and recovery. The JCAHO standards expect that a systematic approach will be taken to provide patient education in institutions.

According to the JCAHO, the goal of patient and family education is to improve patient health outcomes by promoting healthy behaviors and involving the patient in care and care decisions (JCAHO, 2001). This book will only discuss some of the JCAHO goals, processes, and standards. It is important for the nurse who provides patient education to read the entire chapter on Education from the Comprehensive Accreditation Manual for Hospitals (JCAHO, 2001). Box 6-1 lists some of the JCAHO processes for patient and family education.

Joint Commission on the Accreditation of Healthcare Organizations' Standards

There are multiple JCAHO standards that apply to patient education. For the purpose of this book, I have included some of the standards that are applicable to the perinatal setting.

PF.1: The hospital plans for and supports the provision and coordination of patient education activities.

PF.1.1: The hospital identifies and provides the resources necessary for achieving educational objectives.

PF.2: The patient education process is coordinated among appropriate staff or disciplines who are providing care or services.

PF.3: The patient receives education and training specific to the patient's assessed needs, abilities, learning preferences, and readiness to learn as appropriate to the care and services provided by the hospital.

PF.3.1: Based on assessed needs, the patient is educated about how to safely and effectively use medications, according to law and regulation, and the hospital's scope of services, as appropriate.

PF.3.2: The patient is educated about nutritional interventions, modified diets, or oral health, when applicable.

PF.3.4: Patients are educated about pain and managing pain as a part of treatment, as indicated.

PF.3.6: The patient is educated about other available resources and when necessary, how to obtain further care, services, or treatment, as appropriate.

PF.3.7: Education includes information about patient responsibilities in the patient's care.

PF.3.8: Education includes self-care activities, as appropriate.

BOX 6-1

Overview of Some of the JCAHO Processes for Patient and Family Education

Promoting interactive communication between patients and providers

Improving patients' understanding of their health status, options for treatment, and the anticipated risks and benefits of treatment

Encouraging patient participation in decision making about care

Increasing the likelihood that patients will follow their therapeutic plans of care

Maximizing patient self-care skills

Increasing the patients' ability to cope with their health status

Enhancing patient participation in continuing care

Promoting healthy lifestyles

Informing patients about their financial responsibilities for treatment when known (JCAHO, 2001)

PF.3.9: Discharge instructions are given to the patient and those responsible for providing continuing care (JCAHO, 2001).

Providing Patient Education Isn't Easy, Yet We Do It

Nurses face many barriers in attempting to provide quality patient education. No matter the setting, time is a major barrier, because nurses are increasingly caring for patients with higher acuity levels, there are fewer nurses caring for more patients, and the burden of documentation has continued to grow for nurses practicing in both the outpatient and the inpatient arenas. Despite lack of time, nurses still educate patients. We consider it our duty and move forward. In the mother/baby setting, care paths have been used to ensure that essential topics are taught before discharge. In the prenatal care setting, nurses have added subjects formerly taught on postpartum units, such as breast-feeding basics and newborn care, into prenatal classes to be sure that women have an opportunity to learn. Labor and delivery nurses spend precious time teaching women in their triage units about symptoms of preeclampsia or preterm labor, hoping to help the women avert a disaster. No matter the obstacles placed in their way, nurses always teach.

Another barrier to effective patient education is the feeling expressed by some nurses that patient-education activities are not acknowledged as important by the institutions for which they work and that time spent teaching is not rewarded. This is not new but needs to be addressed. Because we as nurses know that patient education is a vital function, it is up to us to help the organizations for which we work understand this. One group of nurses that faced these problems has documented how it forced its institution to notice the results of its patient education efforts (Joseph & Freda, 2001). Those nurses were feeling frustrated and unappreciated by their administration and knew that the time they were spending educating their patients was time well spent, despite the fact that no one seemed to notice the good they were doing. They were being told that the primary care clinic must enroll additional patients, and they intuitively knew they were helping in that effort through teaching the patients who were already enrolled but had no solid evidence of that. They started an organized project, documenting the health histories and patient education they offered to their primary care patients and also documenting the health histories of their patients' families. The nurses assessed the patients' and the patients' families' needs for additional health care and assisted them in making appointments for needed care both for themselves and for their family members. They also called the patients after their visits to determine if the referral appointments had been kept and to offer any other patient education the patients might need. After teaching 50 patients in this new formal way about their health and the health of their families, they checked their results and found that they had added an additional 259 kept appointments to their primary care site! Although the nurses began this project feeling underappreciated for their patient education efforts, they finished it and were lauded by their administration, their colleagues, and their patients. Patient education can make a difference, but nurses must structure their teaching in such a way that institutions and others know the important and essential work that is being done.

In my estimation, it is fortunate for nursing that JCAHO has now made institutions more aware of and accountable for health teaching.

This legitimization of patient education as an integral component of comprehensive care can only be positive for nursing, the profession that has traditionally called patient education its own. Our next step has to be lobbying for third-party reimbursement for patient education. When patient education becomes a reimbursable item, we will have finally gained the legitimacy we so deserve as patient educators.

Prenatal Settings

In the prenatal setting, the provision of comprehensive teaching during pregnancy is not easily accomplished. In some offices or clinics where there are few registered nurses (RNs), whatever patient education occurs is left to the provider of care, who must also administer all of the physical care as well as the education in the time allotted for each visit. This burden is a difficult one to carry alone, especially when the providers of care are physicians, because we know from research that there is a lack of congruence between what physicians believe their prenatal patients want to learn about pregnancy and what the patients themselves want to learn. One study I did with my colleagues (Freda, Andersen, Damus, & Merkatz, 1993a) examined the differences in what pregnant women wanted to know during pregnancy compared with what their physicians believed their patients wanted to know. The study showed a big difference between the perceptions of the patients and the physicians (I bet you're not surprised at that!). For example, the doctors believed their patients wanted to learn about the effect of substance use in pregnancy, but the patients expressed very little interest in this topic. The patients wanted to learn about the use of forceps during childbirth, while the physicians did not believe this topic would be of interest to their patients at all. Another important finding was that all the women wanted to know about fetal growth and development. This was the number one item of interest. This is really important information, because we can use it to help women learn about other essential issues. If we want women to know about a topic in which they have expressed little interest, for instance, we can insert that teaching point in a discussion about fetal growth and development. Because fetal growth and development is interesting to women, the teaching session becomes a win-win situation. The women will be interested because we're talking about fetal growth, and we are able to teach them important information (such as the effects of substance use) that has an effect on fetal growth.

One interesting and innovative method of providing prenatal care and patient education is the "Centering Pregnancy" movement. Begun by Sharon Schindler Rising, CNM, this creative program not only delivers patient education to pregnant women but also delivers prenatal care in an entirely new manner, through working with women in groups instead of individually. It "abolishes routine prenatal care by bringing women out of examination rooms and into groups of 8–12 . . . they meet for 10 ninety-minute visits during pregnancy, during which an educational format is followed with discussions, and the women are encouraged to take responsibility for themselves, thus shifting the patient-provider power base" (Rising, 1998, www.centeringpregnancy.com).

Innovative, creative programs such as this that tackle the problems of helping women learn during the prenatal period, are exciting new developments in the world of patient education.

Intrapartum Settings

In the intrapartum setting, nurses are continually educating their patients, despite the many barriers to effective patient education that exist. Chief among these barriers is that fact that intrapartum nurses are often caring for several patients at the same time and rarely have quality written health education materials to give to their patients. Also, during the intrapartum period the patient is appropriately concentrating on her labor experience. The nurse functioning in this intimate atmosphere with laboring women has unique opportunities to teach her patient and the family about anatomy and physiology, the biology of reproduction, the science of labor management, the procedures being carried out in the labor and delivery (L&D) unit, and about labor and birth itself. Intrapartum nurses are also instrumental in the choices laboring women make during labor, including analgesia, anesthesia, and breast-feeding. It is a powerful role, occurring at a most vulnerable and needy time in a family's life.

Nurses who work in triage units contained in L&D have many opportunities to teach their patients as well. Patients especially in need of education are those who will be going home after a period of triage. Teaching about signs of preeclampsia, signs of preterm labor, and other danger signals is common. Unfortunately, L&D nurses rarely have access to appropriate health education materials for their patients, despite all the teaching they do. This book, however, contains many teaching handouts that L&D nurses can use daily for their patients.

Postpartum and Mother/Baby Settings

In the postpartum or mother/baby setting, patient education is mandated, yet it is difficult to accomplish due to time constraints. Nurses on these units often make use of care paths to accomplish the required teaching in a short period of time. Mother/baby nurses continue to offer group classes to new mothers to teach newborn care, despite the shortened length of stay in hospitals or birthing centers. Some hospitals and birthing centers offer postpartum education via closed-circuit television, using commercial videotapes about commonly needed topics. Although this would seem to meet the needs of administrators to say that patient education has been offered, the effectiveness of these closed-circuit television educational models has not been scientifically evaluated. We have no evidence about whether they actually help new mothers learn important topics.

Although mother/baby nurses might have more access to written materials and videotapes, the shortened length of stay has made their job of educating new mothers a difficult one indeed.

Home Care Settings

Nurses such as public health nurses who make home visits to pregnant or postpartum women also face barriers to effective patient education but consider the education of their patients one of their primary duties. The home environment itself can be a barrier because of the many distractions in the home. The woman might be caring for children other than the newborn, or she might be living in suboptimal conditions. In addition, public health nurses are also expected to make a certain number visits each day and may not have the amount of time they would ideally like to have to teach the woman.

Nurses who visit women at home, however, often have advantages as well. The privacy that might be available in a home setting lends itself well to the discussion of intimate issues. In addition, the nurse who sees the woman's living conditions is able to understand the context of the woman's life. The nurse might then be better able

to realistically assess the woman's ability to comply with instructions or conversely to understand why the woman has been unable to change her behavior.

Assessing What the Patient Needs to Know

The first step in being a good patient educator, no matter what perinatal area you work in, is assessing what the patient needs to know.

In every circumstance when you have the impulse to teach, always begin by asking the woman what she already knows about the topic and assessing what she needs to know, as well as what she wants to know. Don't just teach her what <u>you</u> think she should know.

For example, you might choose to teach a lesson on the effect of smoking during pregnancy, but during the lecture you find that the patient is uninterested. She is looking around the room, going through her handbag, or staring into space. Why? Perhaps she is bored. Perhaps if you had asked her what she knows about the subject before you began the class, you would have learned that she stopped smoking months before she became pregnant and already knows a great deal about this topic. What a shame that you have then used the precious time you have for teaching to teach something your patient doesn't need! There are probably many other topics she needs to learn, but unless you assess her needs, you won't know how to proceed.

A Needs Assessment Survey

Perhaps you already have a needs assessment learning tool for pregnant women. If you have one, use it. Women can complete such a tool while waiting to be seen or during their time with you. There are many different tools to use. Box 6-2 provides an example of just one needs assessment for pregnancy learning.

After Your Needs Assessment, What Then?

After you have assessed what your patients need and want to learn, it is time to plan your teaching. What is your usual method of teaching your patients? Do you provide all the information yourself, one-on-one? Do you use written handouts, films, videotape, or computer-assisted pro-

---

BOX 6-2

Sample Needs Assessment Tool

This is a list of some important topics for you to learn about during pregnancy. Please make a check mark next to all the topics you want to learn about.

_____ Your Rights and Responsibilities During Pregnancy	_____ Circumcision
_____ Fetal Growth and Development	_____ "Natural Childbirth"
_____ Why Is Prenatal Care So Important?	_____ Your Rights and Responsibilities in Labor
_____ Screening Tests in Pregnancy	_____ Cesarean Birth
_____ Smoking and Its Effects	_____ Vaginal Birth After Cesarean
_____ Drug Use and Its Effects	_____ What is a Doula?
_____ Domestic Violence	_____ Hospital Visiting Policies
_____ Nutrition in Pregnancy	_____ Your Hospital Stay After You Give Birth
_____ Fetal Movement Counting	_____ Mother/Baby Care in the Hospital
_____ Sexually Transmitted Diseases	_____ What is "Rooming In?"
_____ HIV Testing and Why It Is Important	_____ Postpartum Blues & Depression
_____ in Pregnancy	_____ Breast-feeding
_____ Ultrasounds, NSTs, Biophysical Profiles	_____ Bottle-feeding
_____ Warning Signs in Pregnancy	_____ Do You Need Home Care?
_____ How to Cope With Bedrest	_____ Getting the Help You Need at Home
_____ Preterm Labor Symptoms	_____ Getting Back to "Normal"
_____ High-Risk Conditions in Pregnancy	_____ Baby Care
_____ Twins or More	_____ Diapering
_____ Questions to Ask Your Provider About Labor	_____ Danger Signs About Newborn Health
_____ When to Come to the Hospital	_____ How Long Should Babies Sleep?
_____ What to Bring to the Hospital	_____ How to Take Your Baby's Temperature
_____ Pain Relief in Labor	_____ Bathing Your Baby
_____ What to Expect in Labor	_____ Spoiling and Other Myths
_____ Electronic Fetal Monitoring	_____ Family Planning
_____ Hydrotherapy (Water Tubs) in Labor	

---

gram information? Are your written or audiovisual materials appropriate for the women in your population? Do you include the family in the teaching? Do you teach the woman in a group setting, along with other women experiencing the same diagnosis? Is there one "best method" for providing patient education?

There is no one method of providing patient education that has been found to be superior to any other.

Individual teaching, group teaching, videotapes for teaching, and computer-aided teaching are all effective but are most effective when chosen for the appropriate patient, with the appropriate diagnosis, using the appropriate materials (Freda, Andersen, Damus, Poust, Brustman, & Merkatz, 1990; Freda, Damus, & Merkatz, 1991; Freeman & Orlandi, 1997; Leff, 1988; Lindeman, 1988; Long, 1992; Mullen, Ramirez, & Groff,

1994; Mullen, Green, & Persinger, 1985; O'Donnell, San Doval, Duran, O'Donnell, 1995; Padgett, 1988; Theis & Johnson, 1995; Tomaino-Brunner, Freda, Damus, & Runowicz, 1998). No matter which method is chosen, however, the principles of adult learning need to be kept in mind. All patient education should be planned to meet the individual learner's abilities, using the most appropriate personnel and materials, and always should be interactive.

One-on-One Teaching

The most commonly used method of teaching pregnant women is one-on-one education, in which the provider teaches the woman about one particular topic in the midst of an encounter in an office, a clinic, or a hospital visit. This method is effective in increasing knowledge and promoting behavior change and is optimally performed by a knowledgeable provider who uses the principles of patient education to inform the teaching (Redman, 1997). One-on-one teaching is especially appropriate when sensitive or private topics need to be discussed. Nurses who wish to teach women about how to disclose HIV-positive status to a loved one, for instance, might appropriately choose individual one-to-one teaching with role-playing rather than assembling a group of similar women for instruction. In addition, for a simple concept, such as teaching fetal movement counting, it has been shown that teaching women this skill within the context of an obstetrical visit is effective not only in promoting the counting of fetal movements but also has the added benefit of increasing maternal–fetal attachment, which fosters positive postpartum attachment behaviors (Bloom,1995; Freda, Mikhail, Polizzotto, Mazloom, & Merkatz, 1993; Mikhail et al., 1991).

The major disadvantage of one-on-one teaching is that it is not cost-effective, because it is the most time-consuming method for the provider (Redman, 1997). When pregnancy-related topics must be taught often to many women, more cost-effective methods, such as group classes, should be considered. Because one-on-one teaching is the method most often used in private offices, it is also instructive to consider whether that methodology results in comprehensive education during pregnancy. In one study that examined the difference between what private care and public care patients were taught in pregnancy, it was found that the public care patients were taught a greater variety of pregnancy-related topics. Because public care settings generally offer more group teaching opportunities than private office settings, these results suggest that we should re-think the customary methodology of teaching women on a one-on-one basis and consider putting in place more cost-effective methods that more effectively educate pregnant women about topics of importance in pregnancy (Freda, Andersen, Damus, & Merkatz, 1993b).

If your practice setting demands one-on-one teaching, there are several things you can do to ensure that the teaching is most effective.

How to Deliver Effective One-on-One Patient Education

- First, assess the woman's learning needs. Ask her what she knows about the topic that you intend to teach before you begin teaching. If she indeed already knows what she needs to know, you can feel comfortable moving on to the next topic.

- Second, don't overteach. As explained in Chapter 1, choose the three or four most important things for the woman to know, and then teach those items. Use an appropriate videotape for the teaching if possible, and then ask the woman to explain what she saw and heard.

- Third, always ask the woman to restate what you have taught. This is your opportunity to correct misconceptions.

- Fourth, always use a handout written at the appropriate readability level during the teaching, and give the handout to the woman to take home. This can reinforce what you've taught.

Group Teaching

For most topics of interest to pregnant women, group teaching of patients costs less than one-on-one teaching and is very effective (Leff, 1988; Likar, Panciera, Erickson, & Rounds, 1997). Studies done with women being taught about preterm labor symptoms, diabetes management, contraception, smoking cessation, parenting, breast-feeding, and childbirth preparation all detail increased knowledge and behavior change when women are taught in groups (Freda et al., 1991; Freda, Damus, Andersen, & Merkatz, 1990; Gagliardino & Etchegoyen, 2001; Hobel, 1994; Jones, 1986; Koniak-Griffin, Verzemnieks, & Cahill, 1992; Mullen et al., 1994; Lowe, 1991; Waller, Zollinger, Saywell, & Kubisty, 1996). Registered nurses are the obvious choice as teachers of groups of pregnant women, because nurses are the health professionals who consider patient education an integral part of their professional duties. The use of RNs for patient education is seen often in public care settings and in some health maintenance organizations (HMOs), but is increasingly apparent in multi-physician private practices. Some of the additional advantages of group teaching include the availability of support from the other group members, questions asked by group members that might not have been considered by each individual patient, and the modeling of behaviors and skills by the teacher and by the group members. Group teaching is best done for general topics of interest to most patients. Early prenatal care education, for instance, includes nutrition education, genetic screening tests, and common discomforts of pregnancy, which are topics often covered in group instruction (Freda, Andersen et al., 1990; Freda et al., 1998; Lindeman, 1988). Childbirth education classes are a classic example of group learning. Fortunately, these classes have become a routine part of pregnancy care for a substantial number of women in the United States.

Should You Offer Group Classes?

Where do you start if you want to develop group teaching classes? First you need to think "outside the box," and recall what you've read in this book. Even if every group class you've ever seen has been in a lecture format, you should think of a better way to teach the women you serve. Group classes cannot, and actually should not, always be in the lecture format so familiar to all of us. Remembering the Adult Learning Principles from Chapter 2, adult learners learn best when their **educational sessions are interactive**. The lecture format puts people to sleep! Box 6-3 describes some tips for group teaching.

In deciding if you should begin group classes, it is essential that you assess the needs and desires of the women in the setting in which you work. Not every population of women will be interested in coming for educational classes. For some women, using reading materials might be just what they want. For others, videotapes at home might be the best way to learn. For others, group classes during which they can talk to other women and get answers to their questions might be the best way for them to learn. Still others don't enjoy groups and will want to talk to you in private about all their questions. We can't assume that all women want to learn in the same way.

How Do You Decide What Type of Education to Offer?

How do you assess whether your population wants group classes? You could develop a short survey and distribute it for a whole week to everyone who comes for care, and then evaluate the answers. What kind of things do you want to ask? For example, your survey might look something like the survey shown in Box 6-4.

BOX 6-3
Some Tips for Group Classes

- Have the women introduce themselves to each other.

- Get a dialogue going between the women about their birth experiences.

- Ask the women what they know about the topic at hand.

- Ask the women if there is anything special they want to know about the topic (if they have questions they want answered, they might not be able to listen effectively during the session).

- Use media such as videotapes.

- Encourage the women to take notes during the media presentation.

- Stay in the room during the media presentation—it says that you are interested.

- Provide healthy snacks and drinks.

- Be sure the seats are comfortable and the room is not too hot or cold.

- Keep the group interactive—don't lecture.

- Ask questions and ask for comments from the group.

- Be a facilitator of knowledge, answering questions and correcting misconceptions, rather than a lecturer.

- Use a hands-on approach whenever possible; don't just demonstrate a skill. When practicing the baby bath, for instance, help the women to bathe their own babies or dolls.

- Before the group session ends, be sure to ask the group if all of their questions have been answered.

BOX 6-4

Sample Survey for Developing Patient Education Programs

How old are you?_____

How many pregnancies have you had in the past? _____ none _____ 1 _____ more than one

1. How are you learning what you want to know about pregnancy and birth? Please choose all the answers that are right for you.

_____ From my provider _____ From the nurse _____ From my family

_____ From my friends _____ From books and magazines

_____ Other (please describe)_____

2. Do you feel that you are learning as much as you need to know?

_____ Yes _____ No _____ Not sure

3. Would you like to have a more formal way of learning about pregnancy as a part of your prenatal care from the nurses in this office/clinic?

_____ Yes _____ No _____ Not sure

4. If you were offered a series of educational sessions about pregnancy, would you be interested in attending?

_____ Yes _____ No _____ Not sure

5. When would be the best time for you to go to a 1-hour class?

_____ Mornings _____ Afternoons _____ Evenings
_____ Weekends

6. What special topics would you like the nurses to include in these classes?

_____

_____

7. If we could arrange it, would you enjoy having a "lending library" of educational videotapes available to you as a part of your pregnancy care?

_____ Yes _____ No _____ Not sure

After collecting the surveys for about a week, you should have a good idea of what your particular population thinks about formal group classes for pregnant women. Some populations will enjoy them, whereas some may not. It is certainly best for you to understand what the population you work with desires before setting up a program that might not be successful.

If your population overwhelmingly enjoys reading materials about pregnancy rather than formal classes, you could develop a listing of the best reading materials, and then spend time at each visit discussing those reading materials with the women. If your population expresses no interest in separate classes given apart from their prenatal visits, it might be best for you to develop group classes **during prenatal care sessions as a part of the prenatal care visit**. When planning something such as this, "outside-the-box" thinking is important. Prenatal care visits have traditionally been 15 minutes in length (due to the fact that only minimal interventions are done each time) but it doesn't have to be that way. Remember that the Expert Panel on the Content of Prenatal Care has suggested that every prenatal care visit should be an educational visit (U.S. Public Health Service, 1989). This will require creative scheduling on your part. Perhaps classes can be scheduled so that all the women who come between 9 AM. and noon will also be scheduled to see two educational videotapes **as a part of each visit.** The women would not just sit in the waiting room when they arrive. They could be shown into the video room several at a time (depending on the size of the practice), watch videotapes chosen by you, discuss the videos, and then see the provider. You can function as the facilitator for those videotaped educational sessions, asking the women questions about what they learned and answering the questions the women have.

If you set up a system such as this, it is essential that the providers of care (nurse practitioners, midwives, physicians) be a part of the plan, because everyone must agree that the educational part of the visit is as important as the physical examination and laboratory testing. If providers feel that the education is "extra," women could get the message that they are just seeing videotapes as a way of "killing time" when waiting for the provider. Nothing could be farther from the truth. Everyone in the practice must be on board with integrating formal education into the prenatal care visit.

Videotape Teaching

In recent years, we have witnessed the proliferation of the videotape used as a methodology for many educational programs, and patient education is no exception (Brown, 1990; Freda, Damus, et al., 1990; Healton & Messeri, 1993; Long, 1992; O'Donnell, San Doval, Vornfett, & DeJong, 1994). There are many reasons for this proliferation, including that our entire society has become used to visual images for learning as well as for entertainment through television, videotapes, and computers. There are numerous companies that produce such videotapes. Use of videotapes has been found to be an effective method of delivering standardized information to patients during individual or group teaching sessions and is especially helpful for low literacy populations (Callahan & Chan, 2001; Freda et al., 1994; Thomas, Daly, Perryman, & Stockton, 2000; Williams, Wolgin, & Hodge, 1998). There are certain caveats that should be kept in mind when using this methodology (Box 6-5).

Videotaped patient education can be a powerful learning tool. It has been shown to be more effective, however, when followed by facilitation by a nurse who can clarify information and answer questions than when used as a stand-alone method of teaching. There is research to support this. In O'Donnell et al.'s (1995) study, videotaped information with an imbedded suggestion for obtaining coupons and redeeming them was used for teaching sexually transmitted disease (STD) prevention. When a videotape alone was used for teaching, 27.6% of the patients used the information to redeem coupons. When facilitation with a provider answering questions was furnished after the videotape, 36.9% of the patients used the information. When just oral teaching without a videotape was used, 21.2% of the patients redeemed

BOX 6-5

Some Ideas for the Best Use of Audiovisual Materials

- Audiovisual materials, such as videotapes, should be no longer than 11–15 minutes, because information presented after that time period is not retained well.

- If you want to use videotapes, and I encourage their use, you should always arrange to preview the videotape before using it for your patients, because it is important that the videotape portray situations and conditions that are culturally relevant to the group that will view it (O'Donnell et al., 1994). Never just purchase a videotape for patient education unless you preview it first. During the preview process, you should also be cognizant of the language used in the videotape and determine if the literacy level is appropriate for the designated population. Videotapes made by commercial companies often have advertisements for the products in the tape. Be sure you check for this and decide if this is what you want your patients to see.

- Be sure that the patients who watch the videotape are seated in a comfortable quiet room. Give them paper and pencils to write down their questions.

- Be the facilitator of learning after the videotape is over. Ask the patients what they learned, and answer all the questions they have. Never use a videotape as a substitute for your personal interaction with the patients.

coupons. These differences were statistically significant (O'Donnell et al., 1995).

What About Showing Videotapes in Waiting Rooms?

In recent years there has been an expansion of videotaped educational programs being shown in waiting rooms of clinics and private offices, with the express intention of teaching patients through this methodology. My colleagues and I studied this phenomenon, because it concerned us that providers would think they no longer needed to teach in person. In our study, the use of "passive" waiting room teaching with videotapes was found to be ineffective in teaching the women most in need of quality patient education—primiparas, African American women, and pregnant women under the age of 20 (Freda et al., 1994). We concluded, and continue to conclude, that videotapes shown in waiting rooms should always be considered an adjunct to enhance patient education, not a methodology unto itself. It might seem that showing educational videotapes in a waiting room is better than having soap operas being shown, but women actually spend very little time watching educational videotapes in a busy, noisy waiting room, and the educational messages from the videotape can be easily missed.

If, however, there is a separate, quiet area in the waiting room or near the waiting room for videotape education—a special place where the woman can pay attention to the videotape—some learning might take place. That has not been studied yet, but we can guess that it will be more effective than waiting room videotapes shown to a general group of people, only some of whom might be interested, or even watching.

Computers for Patient Education

Computers are being used for patient education in a variety of ways. Pregnant women use computers in their homes to access information formerly not available to them, and nurses use computers not only to design health education materials for their patients but also as an adjunct to structured health education classes.

Computer-Aided Instruction for Patients

Computer-aided instruction, or CAI, is used by some patient educators (Consoli, Ben Said, Jean, Menard, Plouin, & Chatelier, 1995; Skinner, Siegfried, Kegler, & Strecher, 1993; Tronni & Wele-

bob, 1996). CAI patient education is that which the patient uses by sitting at a computer and interacting with a specific program that was designed to teach the patient something about health or illness. That program can be one the patient purchases, such as a CD-ROM or a DVD, or one that is a part of an Internet health site. Many computer programs developed for patient education have been didactic, with little or no tailoring of the material to the specific needs of the individual patient. Very few have been evaluated for effectiveness, although one study that found increased knowledge in patients who used the CAI compared with standard methods of patient education described the importance of the CAI being interactive (asking the patient to answer questions) rather than simply didactic (explaining concepts in a lecture format) in nature (Consoli, Ben Said, Jean, Menard, Plouin, & Chatelier, 1996).

As the use of computers for patient education increases in the future, we can expect that software companies will be increasingly tapping the market of adults wanting to learn more about pregnancy, especially issues in high-risk pregnancy. We should be remember, however, that as with videotaped information, CAI should not be a replacement for the teacher/learner interaction but rather an enhancer of that interaction. There are many CD-ROMs and DVDs available from educational companies designed to teach pregnant women about what to expect in pregnancy, just as popular books have for decades. It is always a good idea for providers to preview what advice is being proffered in the most popular CD-ROMs, in anticipation of the questions that will be asked by their patients.

Using Your Computer to Design Patient Education Materials

Another important use of computers in patient education is for the development of patient educational materials that can then be tailored to the specific needs of patient population. The widespread use of desktop publishing has made this practice practical for even the small office or home setting. The development of health education materials is not a simple task, however. See Chapter 7 for a complete discussion of this topic.

Using the Internet for Patient Education

For the patient who is familiar with computers and the Internet, there are myriad health education outlets available through the World Wide

Web and its many search engines. Use of the Internet for patient education has been studied, with interesting results. Leaffer and Gonda (2000) studied 100 senior citizens who were taught to use the Internet to retrieve health information and found that all of them were still using the Internet for those purposes 90 days later, and 66% of them were taking the information they found on the Internet to their health care providers when they had a scheduled visit. More than 50% reported that using the Internet made them feel more satisfied with their treatments, because they felt more knowledgeable. The use of the World Wide Web for patient education is a resource about which we know little at present, but that will inevitably have a major impact on what our patients know and how they learn. Not only are there myriad Websites designed specifically for patient education, but for those women who are interested in the latest research findings about any aspect of pregnancy, the National Library of Medicine now provides public access to MEDLINE (http://www.ncbi.nlm.nih.gov/PubMed). This is an essential resource for nurses as well. Interesting and informative sites are being added to the World Wide Web daily and can be found easily by using Yahoo!, Lycos, InfoSeek, or any other search engine provided by the Internet access company used by the patient. A Lycos search using the words "high risk pregnancy," for instance, yielded 4,967 separate sites where information could be gathered on every conceivable aspect of high-risk pregnancy!

The evolution of the World Wide Web as an important source of health information for our patients is an exciting development, because it empowers the patients to find information they would not have had access to in the past. Some Websites are legitimate and offer appropriate information, whereas others offer blatantly incorrect information and simply opinion. **Information on the Internet is not monitored by any regulatory body.** It is essential, therefore, that nurses become computer literate, understand the World Wide Web, and be competent to search the Internet and read and critique what their patients are finding there. According to Lamp & Howard (1999), there are some criteria you can use and teach to your patients to evaluate the legitimacy of Internet sites.

Some Criteria to Evaluate Websites

1. Is the Website affiliated with a university medical school or professional organization?
2. Are the credentials, educational backgrounds, affiliations, or board certifications of those providing the information listed?
3. Is the information referenced to identify the source of the data?
4. Is the date of the most recent posting included?
5. Are extremely positive claims avoided, especially those made by a commercial sponsor?
6. Is the site easily accessible, easy to use, and easy to read? (Lamp & Howard, 1999)

Nurses who want to suggest useful World Wide Web sites for their patients should first review multiple Websites and use the above criteria to evaluate them. Some Websites that we know to be thorough, accurate, and easy-to-use include the following:

March of Dimes Birth Defects Foundation (http://www.modimes.org)

Baby Center (http://www.babycenter.com)

Family Education Network (http://www.familyeducation.com)

The National Fathering Center (http://www. fathers.com)

Healthfinder (http://www.healthfinder.gov)

WebMD (http://www.webmd.com)

Pampers Parenting Institute (http://www.pampers.com), (in the interest of full disclosure, this is a site for which I write some "Ask the Expert" answers for pregnancy)

Lamaze International (http://www.lamaze.com)

Centering Pregnancy (http://www.centeringpregnancy.com)

Websites Change Often!

It is also important for you to know that Websites change. Sometimes the ownership changes, sometimes the address changes, and sometimes the reliability of the content changes if the site was sold or is under new management. Looking at a Website once today will not tell you how reliable it will be 6 months from now. Therefore, I can only say that the above-mentioned Websites met standards for reliability just before this book was published. Before you choose to recommend any of them (or others) to your patients, you should access them and review them yourself.

The following chapter describes how you can learn to develop health education materials and evaluate their effectiveness.

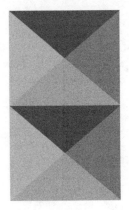

Development and Evaluation of Health Education Materials

I hope this book will provide you with a solid base of patient education materials for your patients, but perhaps your patients have some educational needs not addressed by the materials in this book or in other materials you have been able to locate. If so, you might want to develop materials yourself. Developing health education materials is a time-consuming project, however, so don't go into it thinking it's easy! There is a great deal to consider when developing materials. Those things will be covered in this chapter.

Some Ideas to Keep in Mind When You Develop Health Education Materials

- Assess the real need for the material you think you should develop. Ask the women themselves and the providers.

- Keep it short. Choose the three or four most important things about the topic (these are your learning objectives), and then write only about them. Resist the urge to teach everything you know about a topic.

- Keep it simple. Teach the simple concepts about the topic before the complex ones.

- Don't use medical terminology unless no other word can be used! If medical terminology must be used (such as "amniocentesis"), then define it in simple language.

- Use simple language and short sentences.

- Don't use ambiguous words such as "positive" or "negative" when describing test results. The

general public doesn't understand that sometimes we in health care actually mean a bad outcome when we say "positive" (such as "HIV Positive").

- Use concrete terms—don't be vague. Don't say "Further testing will be required," if you mean to say "You need to come back for another test in 6 months."

- Use a font size of 12 points or larger.

- Use a "serif" font such as Times Roman. Serifs are little bars on the bottoms and tops of the letters.

  This is Times Roman font. It is a <u>serif font</u> and has little bars on the tops and bottoms of the letters. That makes it easier on the eyes.

  This is Helvetica font. It is a <u>sans serif</u> font ("sans" is a French word for "without." It has no little bars on the letters).

- Don't type words using all capital letters—they are more difficult to read.

- Use bold type to emphasize important facts.

- Use illustrations or graphics for interest, but don't use childlike illustrations for materials that will be used for adults.

- Use the active voice.

- Use a question-and-answer format.

- Don't take up every space on the page—leave blank space on the page.

- Avoid double negatives (eg, "You should not avoid green vegetables").

- Be culturally competent. Be sure to use words or examples that the patients in your population can relate to. Ask people of the same culture as your patients to read your material and give you feedback before you give it to patients.

■ Use colored paper—it's more interesting for the reader.

■ Check the readability of what you have written. Be sure it is between the 6th- and 8th-grade levels. If it is higher, then go over it carefully, changing polysyllabic words to shorter words. Change all sentences to short declarative sentences. Then check for readability again. You might have to do this several times before the readability grade level is as low as you desire.

■ Always, always pilot the material you write with some patients before you consider it finished. Ask some (maybe 10) patients to read it and then to tell you what they understood about what they read. You'll learn very quickly where your written material was too complex!

Evaluating the Effectiveness of Health Education Materials

It is our obligation not only to teach our patients but also to evaluate the effectiveness of our teaching. I don't expect that working nurses will undertake formal research projects to accomplish this. If you desire to do research, there are many textbooks and courses that can assist you in these endeavors. For the working nurse, however, there are three really important things you can do to test the effectiveness of the health education materials you are using:

1. _Read the content to be sure it is correct._ An article in _MCN: The American Journal of Maternal-Child Nursing_ addressed just this topic. A nurse wanted to teach about breast-feeding and its effect on risk for breast cancer. She wondered about the accuracy of the content in the booklet she was about to give her patient. This prompted her to read the nursing and medical literature on this topic, where she learned that the material in the booklet was not accurate at all. Read her complete article for more information—I think you'll find it very helpful (Sakai, 2001).

2. _Assess the readability_, a task you can accomplish fairly easily based on the directions in Chapter 3.

3. _Ask your patients to read the materials, and then ask the patients to tell you what the materials said._ This is the simplest of evaluation devices,

and strangely the one strategy least used. Once you know that the material can be read by any given person in your population, it is fairly simple to ask individual patients, or even a group of patients (such as a childbirth education group or some other naturally formed group), to tell you what's good or not good about the materials. This is a great learning experience for any nurse interested in patient education. I've done it innumerable times, and I always learn a great deal from the patients. The patients will tell you what they understood and, probably more importantly, what they didn't understand. Then you'll know what should be fixed.

Other Factors to Consider in Evaluating Health Education Materials

Although readability is one of the most basic factors that we should consider when evaluating patient educational materials, it is not the only important factor. If the woman cannot read the material, she certainly cannot understand it or follow its directions. If, however, she does not want to read it—if she isn't inspired by looking at the material to read it—then she won't try to read it at all! Some of the other factors that should be examined in materials we give our patients are included in an evaluation tool called SAM (Suitability Assessment of Materials). SAM, developed by Doak, Doak, and Root (1996), is an instrument that actually gives a score to materials to decide their usefulness. For the purposes of this book, the scoring of each item will not be included. Just understanding the concepts the authors have chosen, which determine the suitability of materials, is helpful to us. For information about scoring the SAM, see Doak, Doak, and Root (1996).

Some of the Factors Included in the Suitability Assessment of Materials (SAM)

Content
Is the purpose evident?
Is the content about behavior changes?
Is the scope limited to the topic at hand?
Is there a summary at the end to tie up loose ends?

Literacy
Is the readability grade level appropriate?
Is the active voice used?

Is the vocabulary appropriate, using common words?

Is the context explained first?

Are subheadings used to guide the learner?

Graphics

Are the graphics purposeful?

Is the type of graphic used appropriate for the audience?

Are the illustrations illustrative of the purpose?

Are lists or tables well explained?

Are there captions on all the graphics?

Layout

Is it easy to follow the flow of information?

Are shadings, arrows, boxes, etc. used to guide the eye?

Is there adequate white space on the page?

Is the type size at least 12 points?

Has the author avoided using all capital letters?

Learning Motivation

Are the learners asked to answer a question, or make a choice, or otherwise be interactive

Are desired behaviors modeled, such as describing a sample menu rather than just listing appropriate foods?

Is the material presented in a way that makes the behavior change seem possible?

Cultural Appropriateness

Are the language and experience of the intended cultural audience appropriate?

Are the cultural images appropriate?

You can use these categories when you're reviewing the health education materials you use for your patients. If your materials meet or exceed the criteria in SAM, you can be reassured that the materials are appropriate.

This next chapter discusses documentation of patient education.

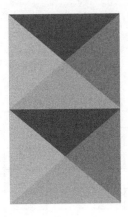

chapter 8

Documenting Patient Education

As nurses we all know how important documentation is. The content of the medical record is the only proof we have of everything we have done for our patients. I know you must remember the same thing I was taught: "If you didn't chart it, it wasn't done." If any of you have ever examined medical records for quality improvement or quality assurance reviews, you understand this concept completely; missing documentation reflects lack of care. Documentation is also required by the Joint Commission on the Accreditation of Healthcare Organizations (JCAHO), is necessary for reimbursement of many services, and is essential for continuity of care so all the health care team members know what has been done for the patients. Additionally, according to Simpson and Chez (2001), the medical record is often the single most important document available in the case of legal action, because even if the nurse can't recall specific events in the care of a patient, evidence from the medical record can defend her actions. Simpson and Chez report that documentation ranks second only to patient monitoring and assessment in nursing-related risk exposure. We all know it's difficult to always remember to document our activities, but for our own safety as well as the safety of the patient, we must remember to do so.

Patient education, as an essential part of our practice, must be documented. Teaching our patients takes a great deal of our time, is offered because we care about the well-being of our patients, and demonstrates to others that we have completed a most important part of clinical care (Abe, Catlin, & Mihara, 2001). What aspects of our teaching should we document? That's easy: all of them. When you help a patient to cough and deep breathe after surgery or to hold a pillow against an abdominal incision when she coughs postoperatively, that's patient education. It should be documented. When you teach a patient with gestational diabetes how to use a syringe and draw up insulin, that should be documented. When you teach a woman with symptoms of preterm labor how to modify her lifestyle, hoping to decrease her symptoms, that's patient education and should be documented. When you discuss risk of sexually transmitted disease with a woman whom you know has several intimate sex partners, that's patient education and should be documented. When you look at patient education in this way, you can see that a great deal of what we do as nurses every day, with every patient we encounter, is patient education.

How Should You Document Your Patient Education?

How should you document your patient education activities? Documentation of patient education should focus on what the patient has learned and can do rather than what the nurse has taught. A note stating, "Patient teaching was done," says nothing about what the patient has learned. Rather, you should document what you taught, whether the patient was able to restate the information, and who was present during the teaching.

The method you use for documenting patient education activities is dependent on the institution for which you work and the policies in place

THE MOUNT SINAI HOSPITAL
NEW YORK, NEW YORK

Date

Name

Sex/DOB

MD/Service

PERINATAL EDUCATIONAL NEEDS ASSESSMENT
LEARNING AND TEACHING RECORD

MOTHER CARE				BABY CARE			
Education and Learning Needs	**Date**	**Method/ Outcome**	**RN Initials**	**Education and Learning Needs**	**Date**	**Method / Outcome**	**RN Initials**
UTERINE HEALING				HANDWASHING			
Bleeding/vaginal discharge				NEWBORN CHARACTERISTICS			
Fundal Massage				Appearance			
				Jaundice			
WOUND CARE/POST-OP CARE				NEWBORN ACTIVITY			
C-Section care				Sleeping			
Perineal/episiotomy care				Crying			
				Tremors			
BREAST CARE				COMFORT CARE			
Nipple care				Swaddling			
Breast Engorgement				Stroking			
Self Breast exam				Cuddling			
NUTRITION				NEWBORN CARE			
Fluid Intake				Bath/ Sponge/Tub			
Diet				Umbilical care			
ELIMINATION				Circumcision care			
Voiding				Diapering			
Flatus/Bowel movement				Nail care			
Hemorrhoids				Dressing			
				ELIMINATION			
MEDICATIONS				Voiding			
				Stooling			
REST/ACTIVITY/EXERCISE				SIGNS OF ILLNESS			
Rest Periods				Temperature taking			
Kegel & Tummy exercise				Dehydration			
Getting in/out of bed				Change in normal behavior			
EMOTIONAL CHANGES				NEWBORN SCREENING			
"The Blues"				Metabolic Screening			
"Ups and Downs"				HIV			
SEXUAL ACTIVITY/				SAFETY AND HEALTH			
CONTRACEPTION				INFANT FEEDING B F			
Resumption of sexual activity				Positioning/Latching on			
Methods				Amount/Length of Feeding			
				Frequency			
Spiritual/Cultural Issue: Date _____				Sucking Patterns			
_____				Breaking Suck			
_____				Burping			
_____				Colostrum/Milk Production			
_____None				Breast Pump			
_____ RN				Milk Storage			
				Supplementing			
				Formula Preparation			

TEACHING METHOD		OUTCOME	
V Verbal Instruction	H Handout	1	Verbalizes Understanding
D Demonstration	* See Progress Notes	2	Return Demonstration
AV AudioVisual	K Have Previous Knowledge	3	No Evidence of Learning

Provided in: English_____   Spanish_____   Other_____

RN INITIAL AND SIGNATURE	RN INITIAL AND SIGNATURE

White-Mother's Record   Yellow-Baby's Record   Pink-Mother's Copy   *TEACHING GUIDELINES ON FILE*

MR-1039 (APP4/97)

Figure 8-1. Sample check-off form (used with permission.).

Mother–Baby Discharge Record

Please go through the following list and check whether you understand each topic or need to know more.

Please read ...*For Moms and Babies* booklet given to you **after** the birth of your baby.

I know this already	Doesn't apply to me	I need to know more		Booklet page #	Mother & family reviewed/ demonstrated
			POSTPARTUM		
			Activity – how much is OK	11	*
			Care of perineum and episiotomy	7,8	*
			Postoperative C-section instructions	9	*
			Signs of postpartum complications	11	*
			Changes in vaginal bleeding, return of my period	7	
			Comfort measures for afterpains, constipation and hemorrhoids	7,9	
			Postpartum "baby blues," depression, hormonal changes	10	
			Postpartum exercises for the first weeks	11	
			How to minimize milk production if I'm not nursing	8	
			BABY CARE		
			What to do if baby is choking or gagging	14	*
			How to do skin care/cord care	14	*
			How to take care of the circumcision or genital area Type: Bell/Gomco	13	*
			How to know if my baby is sick and what to do	21	
			What is jaundice and how to detect it	15	
			Use and cleaning of bulb syringe	14,15	*
			How and when to burp baby	17	
			How to position baby after feeding	17	*
			How to complete and obtain a birth certificate	20,21	
			BREAST-FEEDING		
			I attended Breastfeeding class/watched Breast-feeding video ☐ YES ☐ NO		
			How to position baby for feeding	23	*
			How to get baby to latch onto my nipple properly	23	*
			Removal of baby from my nipple	24	*
			What is the supply and demand concept	23,24	*
			When does breast milk come in	25	
			Implications of supplementing for breast-feeding mothers	24	
			Prevention and comfort measures for sore nipples	24	
			Prevention and comfort measures for engorgement	25	
			How to express milk by hand/breast pump	25	
			BOTTLE FEEDING		
			How and when to feed my baby a bottle	16	*
			Reasons for NOT propping bottles	17	
			What formula should my baby drink	16	
			State Law requires use of infant car seat. I have a baby/infant car seat and know how to use it. ☐ YES ☐ NO		

Discharge weight _____ lb _____ oz
Medications:
Mother: None _____ Prescriptions: _____

Baby: None _____ Prescriptions: _____
Discharge Instructions: _____
_____
_____

Follow-up doctor's appointment:
Mother: Date: _____
Baby: Date: _____
Please call your doctor if you have any questions or concerns.

My discharge instructions have been explained to me and I have received a copy.

Signature: _____

Person receiving infant: _____

Postpartum
Discharge Nurse: _____ Date: _____ Time:_____

Nursery Nurse: _____ Date: _____

White–Mother's Record; **Canary**–Baby's Record; **Pink**–Mother

MOTHER-BABY DISCHARGE RECORD
St. John's Mercy Medical Center/St. Louis, MO

Form 583 (11/93)

PKU (Repeat) Instructions (if necessary): By state law your baby must be tested for these metabolic diseases. Bring your baby to the admitting lab on 2L (next to the escalators) within 3-5 days after discharge. No appointment is necessary. You may come Monday through Friday and Saturday morning. There will be no additional charge. Call 569-6814 for specific hours.

Metabolic Screen (PKU/Thyroid/Galactosemia)
Date: _____ Time: _____   Repeat needed: ☐ YES ☐ NO
                                    (If yes - see instructions above.)

Nurses Signature(s) and Initials	

PATIENT IDENTIFICATION

Figure 8-2. Sample documentation sheet (used with permission.).

there. If, by chance, patient education is not currently being documented formally where you work, now is the time for you to think seriously about implementing an official policy and documentation system for all patient education by nurses. You can choose to develop a special form with the most common education topics already included, so the nurse has to check off which topics were taught, what special circumstances occurred during the teaching, and whether the patient could restate the lesson. An example of just such a check-off form used at Mount Sinai Medical Center in New York is included here as a sample of what could be developed and used in your institution (Fig. 8-1). Also see Figure 8-2 for a sample documentation sheet from St. John's Mercy Medical Center, St. Louis.

If you don't want to use a check-off sheet, you can make patient education a part of your nursing process notes, especially if you use the nursing diagnosis of Knowledge Deficit. In documenting your actions to correct the "knowledge deficit," you will want to document the following:

- an assessment of what the patient knows about the topic
- an assessment of what the patient does not know about the topic
- an assessment of the patient's motivation to learn about the topic
- the learning objectives you developed for teaching
- the methods you used to teach
- the information you taught
- any skills demonstrated to the patient
- the response of the patient to the teaching session
- whether the patient was able to restate the teaching
- the presence of family members at the teaching session

For those nurses who work in settings with computerized charting and databases, the documentation of patient education is usually facilitated by those systems. In computerized charting systems, the documentation is often focused on the patient's mastery of learning objectives, as it should be. No matter how the documentation is accomplished, it should be done in such a manner that anyone who reads the medical record will have a clear understanding of all the patient was taught and what she understood.

Now that you've finished Part 1 of this book, it's time to go to Part 2, which contains the actual patient education handouts for your patients. Feel free to copy them and use them for all your patients, and do let me know how well they work for you. Also let me know if there are other topics not included with this book that would be helpful to you.

Don't tear the handouts out of the book! We've bound the book so there's room for you to put the book on a copy machine and copy the handouts that way. If you tear the handouts from the book, you'll lose your original copy, and then subsequent copies will look blurry.

References

Abe N., Catlin A., & Mihara D. (2001). End of life in the NICU: A study of ventilator withdrawal. *MCN, The American Journal of Maternal Child Nursing. 26*(3), 141–146.

Albright J., deGuzman C., Acebo P., Paiva D., Faulkner M., & Swanson J. (1996). Readability of patient education materials: implications for clinical practice. *Applied Nursing Research, 9,* 139–143.

Andre J. (1993). Commentary: Ethical dimensions of informed consent. *Women's Health Issues, 3,* 24.

Arthur V. A. (1995). Written patient information: A review of the literature. *Journal of Advanced Nursing, 21,* 1081–1086.

Ayello E. A. (1993). A critique of the AHCPR's ``preventing pressure ulcers—a patient's guide'' as a written instructional tool. *Decubitus, 6,* 44–46.

Bandura A., & Adams N. E. (1982). Analysis of self-efficacy theory in behavior change. *Cognitive Therapy and Research, 1,* 287–310.

Beaver K., & Luker K. (1997). Readability of patient information booklets for women with breast cancer. *Patient Education and Counseling, 31,* 95–102.

Becker M. H. (1974). The health belief model as predictor of preventive health behavior. *American Journal of Public Health, 64,* 205–216.

Becker M. H., & Janz N. K. (1985). The health belief model applied to understanding diabetes regimen compliance. *Diabetes Educator, 11,* 41–47.

Blankson M. L., Goldenberg R. L., & Keith B. (1994). Noncompliance of high-risk pregnant women in keeping appointments at an obstetric complications clinic. *Southern Medical Journal, 87,* 634–638.

Bloom K. C. (1995). The development of attachment behaviors in pregnant adolescents. *Nursing Research, 44,* 284–289.

Bowen M. (1978). *Family therapy in clinical practice.* New York: Jason Aronson, Inc.

Braddock C. H., Fihn S. D., Levinson W., Jonsen A. R., & Perlman R. A. (1997). How doctors and patients discuss routine clinical decisions: Informed decision making in the outpatient setting. *Journal of General Internal Medicine, 12,* 339–345.

Brown S. A. (1990). Studies of educational interventions and outcomes in diabetic adults: A meta analysis revisited. *Patient Education and Counseling, 16,* 189–215.

Brownsen K. (1998). Education handouts: Are we wasting our time? *Journal for Nurses in Staff Development, 14*(4), 176.

Cady R. (2000). Informed consent for adults: A review of basic principles. *MCN, The American Journal of Maternal Child Nursing, 25*(2), 106.

Calabro K., Taylor W. C., & Kapadia A. (1996). Pregnancy, alcohol use and the effectiveness of written health education materials. *Patient Education and Counseling, 2,* 301–309.

Callahan P., & Chan H. C. (2001). The effect of videotaped or written information on Chinese gastroscopy patients' clinical outcomes. *Patient Education and Counseling 42*(3), 225–230.

Callister L., Lauri S., & Vehvilainen-Julkunen K. (2000). A description of birth in Finland. *MCN, The American Journal of Maternal Child Nursing, 25*(3), 146–150.

Capitulo K. L., Cornelio M. A., Lenz E. R. (2001). Translating the short version of the perinatal grief scale: Process and challenges. *Applied Nursing Research 14*(3), 165–70.

Charles C., Gafni A., & Whelan T. (1997). Shared decision making in the medical encounter: What does it mean? *Social Science in Medicine, 44*(5), 681–692.

Chervenak F. A., & McCullough L. B. (1990). Clinical guidelines to preventing ethical conflicts between pregnant women and their physicians. *American Journal of Obstetrics and Gynecology, 162,* 303–306.

Consoli S. M., Ben Said M., Jean J., Menard J., Plouin P. F., & Chatellier G. (1995). Benefits of a computer-assisted education program for hypertensive patients compared with standard education tools. *Patient Education and Counseling, 26,* 343–347.

Consoli S. M., Ben Said M., Jean J., Menard J., Plouin P. F., & Chatelier G. (1996). Interactive electronic teaching (ISIS): Has the future started? *Journal of Human Hypertension. 10*(1), S69–S72.

Corrarino J., Freda M. C., Barbara M. (1995). Development of a health education booklet for pregnant women with low literacy skills. *Journal of Perinatal Education, 4,* 23–28.

Davis T. C., Mayeaux E. J., Fredrickson D., Bocchini J. A., Jr, Jackson R. H., & Murphy P.W. (1994). Reading ability of parents compared with reading level of pediatric patient education materials. *Pediatrics, 93*(3), 460–468.

Davis R. (2001). The postpartum experience for southeast Asian women in the United States. *MCN,*

The American Journal of Maternal Child Nursing, 26(4), 208–213.

Davis T. C., Dolan N. C., Ferreira M. R., Tomori C., Green K. W., Sipler A. M., & Bennett C.L. (2001). The role of inadequate health literacy skills in colorectal cancer screening. *Cancer Investigation* 19(2), 193–200.

Doak C., Doak L., & Root J. (1996). *Teaching patients with low literacy skills* (2nd ed.). New York: JB Lippincott Company.

Dowe M. C., Lawrence P. A., CarlsonJ., & Kerseling T. C. (1997). Patients' use of health teaching materials at three readability levels. *Applied Nursing Research, 10*, 86–93.

Earley K. J., Blanco J. D., Prien S., & Willis D. (1991). Patient attitudes toward testing for maternal serum alpha-fetoprotein values when results are false-positive or true-negative. *Southern Medical Journal, 84*, 439–441.

Estey A., Musseau A., & Keenan L. (1994). Patient's understanding of health information: A multihospital comparison. *Patient Education and Counseling, 24*, 73–78.

Faden R. R., Chwalow J., Orel-Crosby E., Holtzman N. A., Chase G. A., & Leonard C. O. (1985). What participants understand about a maternal serum alpha-fetoprotein screening program. *American Journal of Public Health, 75*, 1381–1384.

Foss G. (2001). Maternal sensitivity, posttraumatic stress and acculturation in Vietnamese and Hmong women. *MCN, The American Journal of Maternal Child Nursing, 26*(5), 257–263.

Freda M.C. (2000). Educational interventions for high-risk pregnancies. In W.R. Cohen (Ed.), *Cherry and Merkatz' complications of pregnancy*. Philadelphia: Lippincott Williams & Wilkins.

Freda M. C., Damus K. H., & Merkatz I. R. (1999). An evaluation of the readability of ACOG's patient education pamphlets. *Obstetrics and Gynecology, 93* (5), 771–774.

Freda M. C., DeVore N., Valentine-Adams N., Bombard A., & Merkatz I. R. (1998). Informed consent for MSAFP screening in an inner city population: How informed is it? *Journal of Obstetric, Gynecologic and Neonatal Nursing, 27*(1), 99–105.

Freda M.C. (1997). Cultural competence in patient education. *MCN, The American Journal of Maternal Child Nursing, 22*, 219–220.

Freda M.C. (1995). Arrest, trial and failure. *Journal of Obstetric, Gynecologic and Neonatal Nursing, 24*, 393–394.

Freda M. C., Abruzzo M., Davini D., DeVore N., Damus K., & Merkatz I. R. (1994). Are they watching? Are they learning? Prenatal video education in the waiting room. *The Journal of Perinatal Education, 3*, 20–28.

Freda M. C., Andersen H. F., Damus K. H., & Merkatz I. R. (1993a). What do pregnant women really want to know? A comparison of client and

provider perceptions. *Journal of Obstetric, Gynecologic and Neonatal Nursing, 22*, 237–244.

Freda M. C., Andersen H. F., Damus K. H., & Merkatz I. R. (1993b). Is there a difference in the information being given to private vs. public prenatal patients? *American Journal of Obstetrics and Gynecology, 169*, 155–160.

Freda M. C., Mikhail M., Polizzotto R., Mazloom E., & Merkatz I. R. (1993). Fetal movement counting: Which method? *MCN, The American Journal of Maternal Child Nursing, 18*, 314–321.

Freda M. C., Damus K., & Merkatz I. R. (1991). What do pregnant women know about the prevention of preterm birth? *Journal of Obstetric, Gynecologic and Neonatal Nursing, 20*, 140–45.

Freda M. C., Andersen H. F., Damus K., Poust D., Brustman L., & Merkatz I. R. (1990). Lifestyle modification as an intervention for inner city women at high risk for preterm birth. *Journal of Advanced Nursing, 15*, 364–372.

Freda M. C., Damus K., Andersen H. F., & Merkatz I. R. (1990). A PROPP for the Bronx: Preterm birth prevention education in the inner city. *Obstetrics and Gynecology, 76*, 93–96.

Freeman H. P., & Orlandi M. A. (1997). A self-help smoking cessation program for inner city African Americans: Results from the Harlem Health Connection project. *Health Education and Behavior, 24*, 201–217.

Freud S. (1909). Analysis of a phobia in a five year old boy. *Standard Edition. 10*, 3–152.

Gagliardino J. J., & Etchegoyen G. (2001). A model educational program for people with type 2 diabetes: A cooperative Latin American implementation study. *Diabetes Care, 24*(6), 1001–1007.

Glanville I.K. (2000). Moving toward health oriented patient education (HOPE). *Holistic Nursing Practice, 14*(2), 57.

Grimley D. M., Prochaska J. O, Velicer W. F., & Prochaska G. E. (1996). Contraceptive and condom use adoption and maintenance: A stage paradigm approach. *Health Education Quarterly, 22*, 20–35.

Healton C., Taylor S., Burr C., Dumois A., Lowenstein N., & Kaye J. (1996). The impact of patient education about the effect of zidovudine on HIV perinatal transmission: Knowledge gain, attitudes, and behavioral intent among women with and at risk of HIV. *American Journal of Preventive Medicine, 12*, 47–52.

Healton C. G., & Messeri P. (1993). The effect of video interventions on improving knowledge and treatment compliance in the sexually transmitted disease clinic setting. *Sexually Transmitted Diseases, 20*, 70–76.

Hekkenberg R. J., Irish J. C., Rotstein L. E., Brown D. H., & Gullane P. J. (1997). Informed consent in head and neck surgery: How much do patients actually remember? *Journal of Otolaryngology, 26*, 155–159.

Hobel C.J. (1994). The West Los Angeles Preterm Birth Prevention Project. *American Journal of Obstetrics and Gynecology, 170*, 54–62.

Janz N. K., & Becker M. H. (1984). The health belief model, a decade later. *Health Education Quarterly, 11*, 1–47.

Jiminez S.L. (1994). Evaluating the readability of written patient education materials. *The Journal of Perinatal Education, 3*, 188–193.

Joint Commission on the Accreditation of Healthcare Organizations. (2001). Education of the patient: Standards and scoring guidelines. In *2001 comprehensive accreditation manual for hospitals.* Chicago: Author.

Jones M. E., Bond M. L., Gardner S. H., & Hernandez M. C. (2002). A call to action: Acculturation and family planning in Hispanic immigrant women. *MCN, The American Journal of Maternal Child Nursing. 27*(1), 26–32.

Jones L.C. (1986). A meta analysis study of the effects of childbirth education on the parent infant relationship. *Health Care Women International, 7*, 357–370.

Joseph M., & Freda M.C. (2001). The impact of staff nurses in a primary care setting on recruitment of new patients. *The American Journal of Nursing, 101*(2), 26–32.

Kearney M., Murphy S., Irwin K., & Rosenbaum M. (1995). Salvaging self: A grounded theory of pregnancy on crack cocaine. *Nursing Research, 44*, 208–213.

Kearney M. (1997). Drug treatment for women: Traditional models and new directions. *Journal of Obstetric, Gynecologic and Neonatal Nursing, 26*, 459–468.

Klepatsky A., & Mahlmeister L. (1997). Consent and informed consent in perinatal and neonatal settings. *Journal of Perinatal and Neonatal Nursing, 11*, 34–51.

Knowles M. (1980). *The modern practice of adult education.* New York: Cambridge.

Koff E., & Rierdan J. (1995). Early adolescent girls' understanding of menstruation. *Women's Health, 22*, 1–21.

Koniak-Griffin D., Verzemnieks I., & Cahill D. (1992). Using videotaped instruction and feedback to improve adolescents' mothering behaviors. *Journal of Adolescent Health, 13*, 570–575.

Kridli S. (2002). Women's health beliefs and practices among Arab-American women. *MCN, The American Journal of Maternal Child Nursing, 27*(2).

Kuba L.M. (1995). The prenatal testing roller coaster: One mother's story. *The Journal of Perinatal Education, 4*, 19–22.

Lamp J. M., & Howard P. A. (1999). Guiding parents' use of the internet for newborn education. *MCN, The American Journal of Maternal Child Nursing, 24*(1), 33–36.

Leaffer T., & Gonda B. (2000). The Internet: An underutilized tool in patient education. *Computers in Nursing, 18*(1), 47–52.

Leff E. (1988). Comparison of the effectiveness of videotape versus live group infant classes. *Journal of Obstetric, Gynecologic and Neonatal Nursing, 17*, 338–344.

Levinson R.A. (1995). Reproductive and contraceptive knowledge, contraceptive self-efficacy, and contraceptive behavior among teenage women. *Adolescence, 30*, 65–85.

Likar L. L., Panciera T. M., Erickson A. D., & Rounds S. (1997). Group education sessions and compliance with nasal CPAP therapy. *Chest, 111*, 1273–1277.

Lindau S. T., Tomori C., McCarville M. A., & Bennett C. L. (2001). Improving rates of cervical cancer screening and Pap smear follow-up for low income women with limited health literacy. *Cancer Investigation, 19*(3), 316–323.

Lindeman C.A. (1988). Patient education. *Nursing Research, 6*, 29–60.

London F. (1999). *No time to teach? A nurse's guide to patient and family education.* Philadelphia: Lippincott Williams & Wilkins.

Long C. (1992). Teaching parents about infant CPR–lecture or audiovisual tape? *MCN, The American Journal of Maternal Child Nursing, 17*, 30–32.

Lowe N.K. (1991). Maternal confidence in coping with labor: A self-efficacy concept. *Journal of Obstetric, Gynecologic and Neonatal Nursing, 20*, 457–463.

Lurvey L. D., Nager C. W., & Johnson D. D. (1996). Informed consent: A review. *Primary Care Update Ob/Gyn., 3*, 192–196.

Mailloux S. L., Johnson M. E., Fisher D. G., & Pettibone T. J. (1995). How reliable is computerized assessment of readability? *Computers in Nursing. 13*(5), 221–225.

Marteau T. M., Johnston M., Plenicar M., Shaw R., & Slack J. (1988). Development of a self-administered questionnaire to measure women's knowledge of prenatal screening and diagnostic tests. *Journal of Psychosomatic Research, 23*, 403–408.

Marteau T. M., Kidd J., Michie S., Cook R., Johnston M., & Shaw RW. (1993). Anxiety, knowledge and satisfaction in women receiving false positive results on routine prenatal screening: a randomized controlled trial. *Obstetrics and Gynecology, 14*, 185–196.

Mason D. (2001). Promoting health literacy. *American Journal of Nursing, 101*(2), 7.

Maynard A.M. (1999). Preparing readable patient education. *Journal for Nurses in Staff Development, 15*(1), 11–18.

McCartney P. (2000). After birth: Who gets the placenta? *MCN, The American Journal of Maternal Child Nursing, 25*(2), 105.

McFarlane J., & Gondolf E. (1998). Preventing abuse during pregnancy: A clinical protocol. *MCN, The American Journal of Maternal Child Nursing, 23*(1), 22–26.

Meade C. D., & Smith C. F. (1991) Readability formulas: Cautions and criteria. *Patient Education and Counseling, 17*, 153–158.

Meade C. D., & Howser D. M. (1992). Consent forms: How to determine and improve readability. *Oncology Nursing Forum, 19*, 1523–1528.

Meade C., Byrd J., & Lee M. (1989). Improving patient comprehension of literature on smoking. *American Journal of Public Health, 79*, 1411–1412.

Mikhail M., Freda M. C., Merkatz R. B., Polizzotto R., Mazloom E., & Merkatz I. R. (1991). The effect of fetal movement counting on maternal attachment to fetus. *American Journal of Obstetrics and Gynecology, 165*, 988–991.

Moore M. L., & Moos M. K. (2002). Cultural competence in the care of childbearing families. White Plains, NY: March of Dimes.

Mullen P., Ramirez G., & Groff J.Y. (1994). A meta analysis of randomized trials of prenatal smoking cessation interventions. *American Journal of Obstetrics and Gynecology, 171*, 1328–1334.

Mullen P. D., Green L. W., & Persinger G. S. (1985). Clinical trials of patient education for chronic conditions: A comparative meta analysis of intervention types. *Prevention Medicine, 14*, 753–781.

Murphy P. W., Chesson A. L., Berman S. A., Arnold C. L., & Galloway G. (2001). Neurology patient education materials: Do our educational aids fit our patients' needs? *Journal of Neuroscience Nursing, 33*(2), 99–104.

Myhre P. (1996). Myths and facts . . . about how your patient views her diabetes. *Nursing, 26*, 17.

Nightingale F. (1869). *Notes on Nursing.* Philadelphia: J. B. Lippincott Company.

O'Donnell L. N., San Doval A. S., Duran R., & O'Donnell C. (1995). Video-based sexually transmitted disease patient education: Its impact on condom acquisition. *American Journal of Public Health, 85*, 817–822.

O'Donnell L., San Doval A., Vornfett R., & DeJong W. (1994). Reducing AIDS and other STDs among inner city Hispanics: The use of qualitative research in the development of video-based patient education. *AIDS Education and Prevention, 6*, 140–153.

Padgett D. (1988). Meta analysis of the effects of educational and psychoeducational interventions on management of diabetes mellitus. *Journal of Clinical Epidemiology, 41*, 1007–1030.

Pape T. (1997). Legal and ethical considerations of informed consent. *Association of Operating Room Nurses Journal, 65*, 1122–1127.

Prochaska J.O. (1994). The transtheoretical model of change and HIV prevention: A review. *Health Education Quarterly, 21*, 471–486.

Rankin S. H., & Stallings K .D. (2001). *Patient education principles & practice* (4th ed.). Philadelphia: Lippincott Williams & Wilkins.

Readability calculator [Computer software]. (1996). Dallas, TX: Micro Power and Light.

Redman B.K. (1997). *The practice of patient education* (8th ed.). St. Louis: Mosby Year Book, Inc.

Rising S.S. (1998). Centering pregnancy: An interdisciplinary model of empowerment. *Journal of Nurse Midwifery, 43*(1), 46–54.

Saarmann L., Daugherty J., & Riegel B. (2000). Patient teaching to promote behavioral change. *Nursing Outlook, 48*, 281–287.

Sabogal F. (1996). Printed health education materials for diverse communities: suggestions learned from the field. *Health Education Quarterly, 23*, 123–141.

Sakai T. (2001). A short lesson in evidence-based practice: Does breastfeeding reduce risks of breast cancer? *MCN, The American Journal of Maternal Child Nursing, 26*(1), 42–44.

Sandelowski M., & Jones L.C. (1996). Couples' evaluations of foreknowledge of fetal impairment. *Clinical Nursing Research, 5*, 81–96.

Schneiderman, J. (1998). Rituals of placental disposal. *MCN, The American Journal of Maternal Child Nursing. 23*(4), 142–143.

Searight H. R., & Barbarash R. A. (1994). Informed consent: Clinical and legal issues in family practice. *Family Medicine, 26*, 244–249.

Sikkink J. (1990). Patient acceptance of prenatal alpha-fetoprotein screening: A preliminary study. *Family Practice Research Journal, 10*, 123–131.

Simpson K. R., & Chez B. F. (2001). Professional and legal issues. In KR Simpson & P Creehan (Eds.), *AWHONN's perinatal nursing* (2nd ed.). Philadelphia: Lippincott Williams & Wilkins.

Skinner C. S., Siegfried J. C., Kegler M. C., & Strecher V. J. (1993). The potential of computers in patient education. *Patient Education and Counseling, 22*, 27–34.

Theis S. L., & Johnson J. H. (1995). Strategies for teaching patients: A meta analysis. *Clinical Nurse Specialist, 9*, 100–120.

Thomas R., Daly M., Perryman B., & Stockton D. (2000). Forewarned is forearmed–benefits of preparatory information on videocassette for patients receiving chemotherapy or radiotherapy–a randomised controlled trial. *European Journal of Cancer, 36*(12), 1536–1543.

Todd S. J., La Sala K. B., & Neil-Urban S. (2001). An integrated approach to prenatal smoking cessation interventions. *MCN, The American Journal of Maternal Child Nursing, 26*(4), 185–191.

Tomaino-Brunner C., Freda M. C., Damus K., & Runowicz C. D. (1998). Can pre-colposcopy education increase knowledge and decrease anxiety? *Journal of Obstetric, Gynecologic and Neonatal Nursing, 27*(2), 209–213.

Tronni C., & Welebob E. (1996). End-user satisfaction of a patient education tool. *Computers in Nursing, 14*(4), 235–238.

U.S. Public Health Service. (1989). *Caring for our future: The content of prenatal care.* Washington, DC: Author.

Waller C. S., Zollinger T. W., Saywell R. W., & Kubisty K. D. (1996). The Indiana Prenatal Substance Use

Prevention Program: Its impact on smoking cessation among high-risk pregnant women. *Indiana Medicine, 89,* 184–187.

Weiss B. D., & Coyne C. (1997). Communicating with patients who cannot read. *New England Journal of Medicine, 337,* 272–274.

Williams N. H., Wolgin F.; & Hodge C. S. (1998). Creating an educational videotape. *Journal for Nurses in Staff Development, 14*(6), 261–265.

York R., Bhuttarowas P., & Brown L. (1999). The development of nursing in Thailand and its relationship to childbirth practices. *MCN, The American Journal of Maternal Child Nursing, 24*(4), 145–150.

Zion A. B., & Aiman J. (1989). Level of reading difficulty in the American College of Obstetricians and Gynecologists patient education pamphlets. *Obstetrics and Gynecology, 74,* 955–960.

part II

Patient
Education
Handouts

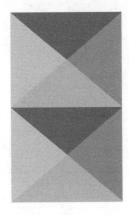

chapter 9

Prenatal Health Education Materials

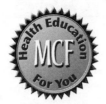

Woman's name: _____

Date: _____

Nurse's name: _____

Choosing a Health Care Provider

General Information

Do you know that in most areas of the United States there are different types of health care providers you can choose to care for you during pregnancy and birth? Perhaps in some very small towns you might have no choice, but you should find out what types of providers are available where you live. It is important that you are comfortable with your provider, and that you and your provider have the same philosophy about pregnancy and birth. The types of providers who usually offer prenatal care and/or birthing services are obstetricians, family practice doctors, nurse practitioners, and certified nurse midwives. The next few handouts discuss the different types of providers.

How Can You Decide What Type of Provider You Should Choose?

- *Ask your friends and family*

    There are some guidelines. First you might ask your friends who have had babies. Who did they use? Were they happy with their choice? Remember, though, that every woman is different. What worked for your friend might not be the best choice for you.

- *What type of birth do you want?*

    Here are some things for you to consider. Before you decide if you want a doctor, a nurse practitioner, or a certified nurse midwife as your provider, you should think about what type of birth experience you want. Some women want a water birth. Some women want their whole family there during the birth. Some women want an epidural for the labor pain. Some women want no medication at all. Some women want to breast-feed right after birth. Some women want to keep their baby with them at all times. Some women want to sleep all night and have the baby kept in a nursery. These are only some of the things you should think about, but they're important. You should try to find a provider who agrees with what you want. Some might not. That might be your clue that perhaps you want a different provider.

- *Reputation counts*

    You should also find a provider who has a good reputation in your community. Unfortunately, not all providers do. Ask questions. Ask your friends, and ask your primary care doctor or nurse. You can even call the state health department in most states to find out if the doctor, nurse, or midwife you are thinking about choosing has a good record and a current license to practice.

- *Which hospital or birthing center do you want?*

    You should also find out which hospitals or birthing centers the doctor, nurse, or midwife is associated with. You might have your heart set on giving birth in Hospital A, but the midwife you want doesn't practice at that hospital. You might be sure that you want to give birth in your local birthing center, with your family all around you, but your family doctor doesn't practice there.

Read the next few handouts to learn the specific things about choosing doctors, nurse practitioners, or midwives for your prenatal care and birth.

Flesch-Kincaid Reading Level: 6.1

Special Instructions _____

Phone number to call if you have questions: _____

Copyright © 2002 Lippincott Williams & Wilkins. Developed by MC Freda, EdD, RN, CHES, FAAN.

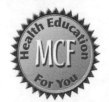

Woman's name: _____

Date: _____

Nurse's name: _____

Eligiendo al Proveedor de Servicios Médicos

Información General

Sabe usted de que en la mayor parte de los Estados Unidos existen varias clases de proveedores de servicios médicos a los que usted puede escoger para su cuidado durante su embarazo y parto. Quizas no tenga ésta opción en algunos pueblos muy pequeños sin embargo, debería de averiguar qué clase de proveedores médicos hay disponibles en su área. Es muy importante de que se sienta cómoda con su proveedor y de que usted y ellos compartan la misma filosofía acerca del embarazo y del parto. Generalmente, las clases de proveedores que ofrecen cuidado prenatal y/o servicios de partos son obstetras, doctores en medicina familiar, enfermeras practicantes, enfermeras comadronas certificadas. Los siguientes folletos explicarán las diferentes clases de proveedores.

¿Cómo puede usted decidir a que clase de proveedor elegir?

- **Pregúntele a sus amistades y familiares**

   Existen algunas pautas. Primero, usted le puede preguntar a sus amistades que hayan tenido bebés. ¿A quiénes utilizaron para el embarazo y el parto? ¿Estubieron satisfechos con su elección? Pero recuerde que cada mujer es diferente. Lo que le funcionó a su amiga puede no ser la mejor selección para usted.

- **¿Qué clase de nacimiento quiere usted?**

   He aquí algunas cosas que debe considerar. Antes de decidir por un doctor, enfermera practicante ó enfermera comadrona certificada como su proveedor, debería de pensar sobre qué clase de experiencia de parto quiere. Algunas mujeres desean partos por agua. Algunas mujeres prefieren que toda su familia estén presente durante el nacimiento. Otras mujeres desean un epidural para el dolor del parto. Algunas mujeres no quieren ninguna clase de medicamento en ningún momento. Algunas mujeres desean amamantar a sus bebés apenas nacen. Otras quieren quedarse con sus bebés todo el tiempo. Otras prefieren dormir toda la noche mientras sus bebés son mantenidos en la guardería infantil. Estas son solamente algunas de las cosas en las que deberta pensar, sin embargo son importantes. Debería de encontrar un proveedor que esté de acuerdo con lo que usted quiere. Algunos no lo pueden estar. Eso puede ser un indicio de que quizás usted necesita otro proveedor.

- **La reputación cuenta**

   Tambien debería encontrar a un proveedor que tenga una buena reputación dentro de su comunidad. Desafortunadamente, no todos son así. Haga preguntas. Pregúntele a sus amistades, y pregúntele a su doctor primario ó enfermera. Inclusive, en la mayoría de los estados usted puede llamar al departamento de salud estatal y averiguar si el doctor enfermera o comadrona que usted está pensando en elegir para su cuidado tienen un buen record o tienen una licencia válida para ejercer.

- **¿Cuál hospital o maternidad desea usted?**

   Ustede debería de averiguar con cuales hospitales o maternidades están afiliados su doctor, enfermera o comadrona. Quizás usted se halla ilusionado en dar a luz en el hospital A, pero la comadrona que usted elegió no practica en ése hospital. Asegúrese de querer dar a luz en su maternidad local, con toda su familia cerca de usted aunque sin embargo su doctor no practique allí.

Lea los siguientes folletos para que comprenda factores específicos sobre como escoger los doctores, enfermeras o comadronas para el cuidado prenatal y parto.

Special Instructions _____

Phone number to call if you have questions: _____

Copyright © 2002 Lippincott Williams & Wilkins. Developed by MC Freda, EdD, RN, CHES, FAAN.

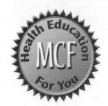

Woman's name: _____

Date: _____

Nurse's name: _____

Choosing a Health Care Provider

Should You Choose a Doctor?

Different Types of Doctors

Obstetrician/Gynecologists

There are two different types of doctors who take care of pregnant women. One type is the Obstetrician/Gynecologist. This is a doctor who has finished medical school and a special 4-year residency program. These doctors only take care of women. They provide prenatal care and do births. They also take care of other women's health problems. The majority of women choose this type of doctor for their prenatal care. Most obstetricians deliver babies at hospitals, although a few do home births. Not all obstetricians believe in the same things, but they are more likely than midwives to use interventions in labor such as fetal monitoring, intravenous fluids, and epidural anesthesia. Women who want these things might want to go to an obstetrician. Be sure to talk to the obstetrician you choose about what you want in labor, so there are no surprises when that time comes.

If you have a chronic illness (such as a heart problem, high blood pressure, thyroid disease, or diabetes) you should probably choose an obstetrician for your pregnancy and birth care. Obstetricians are trained to treat you for all sicknesses you might have before or during a pregnancy.

Family Practice Doctors

Another type of doctor who provides pregnancy and birth care is the family practice doctor. This type of doctor has finished medical school and completed a 3- to 4-year residency in family practice. Family practice doctors are trained to take care of the whole family. Many people enjoy using a doctor who can treat everyone in the family.

If you have a health problem during your pregnancy (such as diabetes), or if you are having twins or triplets, you should probably see an obstetrician for your care. Obstetricians are trained to care for high-risk pregnancies. Family practice doctors do not do surgery. If you needed a Cesarean Birth, an obstetrician would have to be brought in to do it.

Flesch-Kincaid Reading Level: 8.0

Special Instructions _____

_____

_____

Phone number to call if you have questions: _____

Copyright © 2002 Lippincott Williams & Wilkins. Developed by MC Freda, EdD, RN, CHES, FAAN.

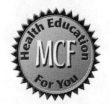

Woman's name: _____
Date: _____
Nurse's name: _____

Eligiendo un Proveedor de Servicios Médicos

¿Debería Usted Escoger a un Doctor?

Diferentes Clases de Doctores

Obstetra/Ginecólogos

Hay dos clases de doctores para el cuidado de las mujeres embarazadas. Uno de ellos es el Ginecólogo/Obstetra. Este es un doctor graduado de la escuela de medicina y un programa especial de residencia de cuatro años . Estos doctores solamente atienden a mujeres. Ellos proveen cuidado prenatal y atienden los partos. También ellos curan otros problemas de salud de las mujeres. La mayoría de las mujeres eligen ésta clase de doctor para su cuidado prenatal. Muchos obstetras atienden los partos de los bebés en los hospitales aunque unos cuantos los atienden en las casas. No todos los obstetras piensan de la misma manera, pero sin embargo ellos estan más dispuestos que las comadronas al uso de intervenciones en los partos tales como el monitor fetal, líquidos intravenosos y anestesia epidural. Las mujeres que deseen éstas cosas deberían de ir donde una obstetra. Asegúrese de conversar con su obstetra acerca de las cosas que usted desea durante el parto para que cuando llegue el momento no se de con sorpresas.

Sí usted tiene una enfermedad crónica (tal como un problema del corazón, presión alta, enfermedad de la tiroides o diabetes) probablemente debería de escoger una obstetra para su embarazo y cuidado natal. Los obstetras estan especialmente entrenados para curar las enfermedades que puedan tener antes o durante un embarazo.

Doctores en Medicina Familiar

Otra clase de doctor que ofrece cuidado del embarazo y natal es el doctor de medicina familiar. Esta clase de doctor ha terminado la escuela de medicina y en tres ó cuatro años ha completado una residencia en medicina familiar. Los doctores en medicina familiar estan entrenados para cuidar a toda la familia. La mayoría de las personas se sienten a gusto al usar un doctor que cuide a toda la familia.

Sí usted tiene un problema de salud durante su embarazo(tal como diabetes o presión alta), o si va a tener mellizos o trillizos, probablemente usted debería de ver una obstetra para su cuidado. Los obstetras estan entrenados para tratar embarazos que tienen alto riesgo. Generalmente, los doctores en medicina familiar no practican cirugía. Sí usted necesita un parto por cesárea, le traeran una obstetra para que lo realice.

Special Instructions _____

_____

_____

Phone number to call if you have questions: _____

Copyright © 2002 Lippincott Williams & Wilkins. Developed by MC Freda, EdD, RN, CHES, FAAN.

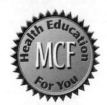

Choosing a Health Care Provider

Should You Choose a Certified Nurse Midwife?

What is a certified nurse midwife?

A certified nurse midwife (CNM) is a Registered Nurse who has completed special training to learn how to care for pregnant women and how to deliver babies. Most CNMs have a master's degree. They take care of about 10% of pregnant women in the United States. They have passed examinations and are licensed by their state both as Registered Nurses and as Certified Nurse Midwives. Their care has been shown to be very safe.

Why would I want to choose a CNM?

CNMs generally have a different philosophy about pregnancy and birth than doctors. Midwives think of pregnancy and birth as normal events for women. Midwives usually spend a lot of time teaching women. They believe in staying with a woman during her labor. They believe in being patient in waiting for the baby to come. They usually take care of women who have normal, healthy pregnancies. If a woman who is being cared for by a midwife becomes sick during pregnancy or in labor, the midwife will call in a doctor. All midwives work with a doctor as a "back-up" for emergencies.

Different types of midwives

There are two different types of midwives. One is the certified nurse midwife and the other is called a "lay midwife." The "lay midwife" is not a nurse, but has been trained (usually by another midwife) to take care of women during pregnancy and birth. Because certified nurse midwives are licensed, you can feel sure that they understand all about prenatal care and birth. Only a few states offer examinations for "lay midwives," however. So, before you choose a midwife for your care, be sure to ask if the midwife is a nurse. If she is not a nurse, ask if she is licensed to practice as a midwife in any state.

Flesch-Kincaid Reading Level: 6.8

Special Instructions _____

_____

_____

_____

Phone number to call if you have questions: _____

Copyright © 2002 Lippincott Williams & Wilkins. Developed by MC Freda, EdD, RN, CHES, FAAN.

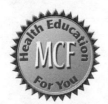

Woman's name: _____
Date: _____
Nurse's name: _____

Eligiendo un Proveedor de Servicios Médicos

¿Debería usted elegir a una enfermera-comadrona certificada?

¿Qué es una enfermera-comadrona certificada?

Una enfermera-comadrona certificada (CNM) es una Enfermera Certificada quién ha completado un entrenamiento especial para aprender cómo cuidar a las mujeres embarazadas y cómo atender los partos. La mayoría de los CNM tienen una maestría. Ellos se encargan de aproximadamente el diez por ciento de las mujeres embarazadas en los Estados Unidos. Ellos han aprobado exámenes y generalmente son acreditados por sus estados como Enfermeras Certificadas y también como Enfermeras-Comadronas Certificadas. Se ha comprobado que su cuidado es muy seguro.

¿Por qué escogería a un CNM?

Generalmente los CNM tienen una filosofía diferente acerca del embarazo y del parto que los doctores. Las comadronas piensan que los embarazos y los partos son cosas normales para las mujeres. Generalmente las comadronas pasan bastante tiempo enseñándole a las mujeres.Creen en acompañar a las mujeres durante sus partos. Creen en tener paciencia en lo que esperan a que nazca el bebé. Generalmente, cuidan a las mujeres que tienen embarazos saludables y normales.Sí, mientras bajo el cuidado de una comadrona, una mujer embarazada se enferma, ella llamará al doctor. En caso de emergencia todas las comadronas trabajan con un doctor en calidad de respaldo.

Diferente clases de comadronas

Hay dos clases de comadronas. Una es la enfermera-comadrona , y la otra "la comadrona no profesional". La "comadrona no professional" no es una enfermera, pero ha sido entrenada (generalmente por otra comadrona) para cuidar a las mujeres durante su embarazo y parto. Debido a que las enfermeras-comadronas certificadas son acreditadas se puede sentir seguro de que ellas comprenden todo lo relacionado con el embarazo y el parto. Solamente unos cuantos estados ofrecen exámenes para las comadronas no profesionales. Así que antes de escoger una comadrona para su cuidado, asegúrese de preguntarle si la comadrona es también una enfermera. Sí no es una enfermera pregúntele si está acreditada para practicar como comadrona en cualquier estado.

Special Instructions _____

_____

_____

Phone number to call if you have questions: _____

Copyright © 2002 Lippincott Williams & Wilkins. Developed by MC Freda, EdD, RN, CHES, FAAN.

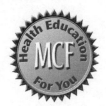

Woman's name: _____

Date: _____

Nurse's name: _____

Choosing a Health Care Provider

Should You Choose a Nurse Practitioner?

What is a Nurse Practitioner?

A nurse practitioner (NP) is a Registered Nurse who has completed special training to learn how to care for pregnant women. Nurse practitioners do not deliver babies; they just take care of women during pregnancy. Nurse practitioners work with certified nurse midwives and with doctors. The midwives or doctors will deliver the baby. Most NPs have a master's degree. They have passed examinations and are licensed by their state as registered nurses and as NPs.

Why Would I Want to Choose a Nurse Practitioner?

Nurse practitioners generally work in doctors' or midwives' offices or in clinics. Although they will not deliver your baby, they can give very good prenatal care. NPs are taught to spend time with the women they take care of and to do a lot of teaching. NPs usually take care of women who have normal healthy pregnancies. If a woman who is being cared for by an NP becomes sick during pregnancy, the NP will call in a doctor.

Flesch-Kincaid Reading Level: 6.9

Special Instructions _____

_____

_____

_____

_____

_____

_____

Phone number to call if you have questions: _____

Copyright © 2002 Lippincott Williams & Wilkins. Developed by MC Freda, EdD, RN, CHES, FAAN.

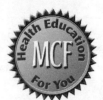

Woman's name: _____

Date: _____

Nurse's name: _____

Eligiendo un Proveedor de Servicios Médicos

¿Debería usted elegir una enfermera titulada?

¿Qué es una Enfermera Titulada?

Una enfermera titulada (NP) es una Enfermera Acreditada quién ha completado un entrenamiento especial para aprender cómo cuidar a las mujeres embarazadas. Las enfermeras tituladas no atienden los partos, pero sin embargo cuidan a las mujeres durante el embarazo.Las enfermeras tituladas trabajan con las enfermeras acreditadas y los doctores. Las comadronas o doctores atienden los partos. La mayoria de las NP's tienen una maestría. Ellas han pasado exámenes y están acreditadas por sus estados, como Enfermeras Acreditadas y como Enfermeras Tituladas.

¿Por qué Quisiera Escoger a una Enfermera Titulada?

Generalmente, las enfermeras tituladas pasan bastante tiempo con las mujeres que cuidan. Usualmente, trabajan en las oficinas de los doctores , comadronas o en clínicas. Aunque ellas no atienden los partos, le pueden brindar un buen cuidado prenatal. NP's están adiestradas para pasar tiempo con las mujeres que cuidan y de ofrecerles mucha enseñanza. Generalmente las NPs cuidan de las mujeres que tienen un embarazo normal y saludable. Si una mujer embarazada se enferma mientras está bajo el cuidado de una NP, ésta llamará a un doctor.

Special Instructions _____

_____

_____

_____

_____

_____

_____

Phone number to call if you have questions: _____

Copyright © 2002 Lippincott Williams & Wilkins. Developed by MC Freda, EdD, RN, CHES, FAAN.

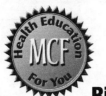

Woman's name: _____

Date: _____

Nurse's name: _____

Rights and Responsibilities of Pregnant Women

Do you know that you have certain rights and responsibilities during pregnancy?

Some of Your Rights

1. You should be told about any **possible risks** of drugs or tests ordered for you or your baby.
2. You should be told if there are **pregnancy education classes** that could help you in labor.
3. You have the right to **make your own decisions** about any tests your doctor, nurse, or midwife wants you to have.
4. You have the right to **know the names** of all the people taking care of you.
5. You have the right to have **someone you care about** with you while you are in labor.
6. You have the right to have a copy of your **medical records**.

Some of Your Responsibilities

1. You are responsible for **learning all you can** about pregnancy so you can make better decisions about what you want.
2. You should find out the **rules of the place where you plan to have your baby** (how to pay, how long you will be there, whether the baby will be in your room, who can visit you, etc.).
3. You should **ask questions** when you don't understand why something is being done.
4. You are responsible for **listening** to your doctor, nurse, or midwife, and deciding what to do after hearing your choices.
5. If you decide to change to a different birth site or provider, you are responsible for **notifying us** so we can send your medical records there.
6. You are responsible for learning all you can about how to **care for your baby at home**.

Adapted from ICEA "The Pregnant Patient's Bill of Rights and Responsibilities."

Flesch-Kincaid Reading Level: 4.8

Special Instructions _____

_____

_____

_____

Phone number to call if you have questions: _____

Copyright © 2002 Lippincott Williams & Wilkins. Developed by MC Freda, EdD, RN, CHES, FAAN.

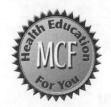

Woman's name: _____
Date: _____
Nurse's name: _____

Derechos Y Responsabilidades De La Mujer Embarazada

¿Sabe que tiene algunos derechos y responsabilidades durante el embarazo?

Algunos De Sus Derechos

1. Se le debe avisar sobre cualquier **riesgo posible** de drogas o pruebas ordenadas para usted o su bebé.
2. Se le debe decir si es que hay algunas **clases de educación del embarazo** que le pueda ayudar con el parto.
3. Tiene el derecho de **hacer sus propias decisiones** sobre las pruebas que su doctor, enfermera o partera quiera que usted se haga.
4. Tiene el derecho de **saber los nombres** de todas las personas que están cuidando de usted.
5. Tiene el derecho de tener a **alguna persona querida** con usted durante su parto.
6. Tiene el derecho de tener una copia de sus **registros médicos**.

Algunas De Sus Responsabilidades

1. Es responsable de **aprendar lo más que pueda** sobre el embarazo para que pueda hacer mejores decisiones sobre lo que desea.
2. Debe aprender **las reglas del lugar donde va a tener a su bebé** (comó pagar, por cuanto tiempo va a estar allí, si el bebé va a estar en su cuarto, quien la puede visitar, etc.).
3. Debe **hacer preguntas** cuando no entienda porque algo se le está haciendo.
4. Es reponsable de **escuchar** a su doctor, enfermera o partera, y decidir después de oir sus opiniones.
5. Si decide cambiar a un lugar diferente de parto o proveedor de salud, es responsable de **notificarnos** para que podamos mandar sus registros médicos a ése lugar.
6. Es responsable de aprender todo lo que pueda sobre el **cuidado de su bebé en casa**.

Adaptado de ICEA "Declaration de Derechos y Responsabilidades del Paciente Embarazad."

Special Instructions _____

_____

_____

_____

Phone number to call if you have questions: _____

Copyright © 2002 Lippincott Williams & Wilkins. Developed by MC Freda, EdD, RN, CHES, FAAN.

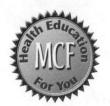

Woman's name: _____

Date: _____

Nurse's name: _____

Why is Prenatal Care So Important?

Now that you're pregnant, your doctor, midwife, or nurse will ask you to come see them often. For most women, prenatal care visits are scheduled each month until the 8th month, then every 2 weeks, and then every week. For some women who have special risk factors, prenatal care visits might be more often.

Why is it important to keep all your prenatal care visits?

Special Tests

Some women think prenatal care is just listening to the baby's heartbeat or checking the mother's blood pressure. Some women think that if they feel okay, it really isn't necessary to go to every prenatal care visit. Those women are wrong. Prenatal care is much more than listening to the baby or checking blood pressure. There are many special tests done during pregnancy that tell us if the baby and the mother are healthy. Some of those tests can **only be done** at certain times in pregnancy. For instance, some pregnant women develop a type of diabetes called "gestational diabetes." If that is not found and treated quickly, both the baby and the mother can become very sick. The test for gestational diabetes needs to be done at a certain time in pregnancy. If you don't come for that visit, we miss an opportunity to be sure you and the baby are well.

There are tests for other pregnancy illnesses that need to be done as well.

Also, there are some infections in pregnancy that you might never know you have unless your provider does a test to find it. Infections can be harmful to you and to the baby.

Health Education

Prenatal care is also important because it's a time for you to learn about your body, what's happening inside you during pregnancy, how your baby is growing, and how to care for yourself and your baby. You should write down all the questions you have at home, and bring that list with you each time you come for a prenatal visit. Your doctor, nurse, or midwife is there for you at each visit so you can ask as many questions as you like. Your provider should also give you some written information (like this) to help you remember what you were taught and to help you learn more.

So, prenatal care is important, and it's best if you keep every visit. Please ask your doctor, nurse, or midwife if you have any questions about what you read here.

Flesch-Kincaid Reading Level: 7.4

Special Instructions _____

_____

Phone number to call if you have questions: _____

Copyright © 2002 Lippincott Williams & Wilkins. Developed by MC Freda, EdD, RN, CHES, FAAN.

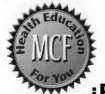

Woman's name: _____

Date: _____

Nurse's name: _____

¿Por qué es tan importante el cuidado prenatal?

Ahora que usted está embarazada, su doctor, comadrona o enfermera le pediran que los visite con más frecuencia. Para la mayoría de las mujeres, las visitas de cuidado prenatal están programadas mensualmente hasta el octavo mes, luego cada dos semanas y posteriormente cada semana. Para algunas mujeres que poseen factores de alto riesgo, las visitas prenatales se harán con más frecuencia

¿Porqué es tan importante acudir a todas sus visitas prenatales?

Exámenes especiales

Algunas mujeres piensan que el cuidado prenatal consiste solamente en escuchar los latidos del bebé, o chequear la presión sanguínea de la madre. Algunas mujeres piensan de que si se sienten bien, no es realmente necesario acudir a cada una de las visitas prenatales. Aquellas mujeres estan equivocadas. El cuidado prenatal es mucho más que escuchar al bebé o chequear la presión sanguínea de la madre. Existen muchos exámenes especiales que se realizan durante el embarazo, lo que nos permiten saber si el bebé o la madre están en perfecta salud. Algunos de esos exámenes **solamente se pueden efectuar durante** ciertas etapas del embarazo. Por ejemplo, algunas mujeres embarazadas desarrollan un tipo de diabetes llamada "diabetes gestacional". Si ésta no es detectada y tratada a tiempo, ambos bebé y madre pueden enfermarse gravemente. La prueba de la diabetes gestacional necesita ser realizada durante cierta etapa del embarazo. Si usted no acude a esta cita, perderemos la oportunidad de asegurarnos que tanto usted como el bebé gozan de buena salud.

Existen otros exámenes para otras enfermedades del embarazo y las cuales tambien se tienen que realizar. Tambien existen otras infecciones del embarazo las cuales usted nunca penso tener, a menos que su proveedor le haga un exámen para así averiguarlo. Las infecciones pueden ser dañinas para tusted y su bebé.

Educación de la Salud

El cuidado prenatal es también importante porque es una oportunidad para que aprenda acerca de su cuerpo, que es lo que está pasando dentro de tu cuerpo durante el embarazo, como se está desarrollando su bebé, y para saber como cuidarse usted y su bebé. En casa usted debería de escribir todas las preguntas que tenga y traer la lista consigo cada vez que acuda a su visita prenatal. Su doctor, enfermera o comadrona están disponibles para que usted les haga todas las preguntas que tenga. Su proveedor debería darle también información por escrito (tal como esta) para ayudarle a recordar lo que se le enseñó, y ayudarle a aprender aún más.

Así que el cuidado prenatal es muy importante, y es mucho mejor si acude a todas sus visitas. Por favor pregúntele a su doctor, enfermera o comadrona cualquier pregunta que tenga sobre lo que ha leído aquí.

Special Instructions _____

_____

Phone number to call if you have questions: _____

Copyright © 2002 Lippincott Williams & Wilkins. Developed by MC Freda, EdD, RN, CHES, FAAN.

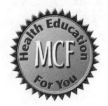

Woman's name: _____

Date: _____

Nurse's name: _____

When Is Your Baby Due?

How Do You Figure Out When Your Baby Is Due?

For most women, it's very exciting to become pregnant and dream about when they will have a new baby. Your doctor, nurse, or midwife will tell you when your baby is due at your first visit, but you can figure this out for yourself! It's really easy!

Think back to the first day of your last menstrual period. Add 7 days to that date. Then subtract 3 months from that date. That will be your due date. Here's an example:

- The first day of your last period was on August 12
- Add 7 days = August 19
- Subtract 3 months = May 19
- May 19 is your due date

Your doctor, nurse, or midwife will call this your EDC, EDD, or EDB. EDC is your "Estimated Date of Confinement" (from the days when women were "confined" when they had babies!). EDD and EDB are the more modern terms, standing for "Estimated Date of Delivery" or "Estimated Date of Birth." Remember that it is an "estimated" date. Very few people actually have their baby on that exact date. It just gives an idea of approximately when your baby will be born. Anything from 2 weeks before that date until 2 weeks after that date is considered normal.

How Long Does A Pregnancy Last?

Most people say that pregnancy lasts 9 months. That's 9 calendar months. Some months have more than 4 weeks in them. Pregnancy lasts about 280 days, or about 40 weeks. Actually, a full-term pregnancy is any pregnancy that lasts from the end of the thirty-seventh week until the end of the forty-second week. If your baby is born before 37 weeks, it will be considered "preterm." If your baby is born after 42 weeks, it will be considered "postterm."

Flesch-Kincaid Reading Level: 4.5

Special Instructions _____

_____

_____

_____

Phone number to call if you have questions: _____

Copyright © 2002 Lippincott Williams & Wilkins. Developed by MC Freda, EdD, RN, CHES, FAAN.

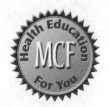

¿Cuándo va a Nacer su Bebé?

¿Cómo Calcular Cuando Va a Nacer su Bebé?

Para la mayoría de las mujeres es muy emocionante el salir embarazada y soñar acerca de cuando tendran su nuevo bebé. Su doctor, enfermera o comadrona le diran en su primera visita, la fecha en que su bebé nacerá, pero sin embargo, usted misma lo puede calcular. ¡Es bien fácil!

Recuérdese la fecha de su última regla. A esa fecha agréguele siete días más. Luego réstele tres meses a partir de esa fecha. Esa será la fecha del nacimiento . He aquí un ejemplo:

- El primer día de su última regla fué agosto 12
- Agregue siete días = agosto 19
- Réstele tres meses = mayo 19
- Su fecha del parto es mayo 19

Su doctor, enfermera o comadrona le llamarán a ésto su FEC, FEP , o FEN. FEC es su : Fecha Estimada de Confinamiento(de la época cuando se confinaban a las mujeres que tenian bebés). FEP y FEN son los términos má modernos, que quieren decir "Fecha Estimada de Parto" o "Fecha Estimada del Nacimiento". Recuerde que ésta es una fecha estimada. Realmente muy pocas personas tienen el bebé en la fecha exacta. Esto sólo nos dá una fecha aproximada de cuando va a nacer el bebé. Se considera normal que el bebé nazca dos semanas antes o dos semanas después de la fecha estimada.

¿Cuánto dura un Embarazo?

La mayoría de las personas dicen que el embarazo dura 9 meses. Esto es 9 meses por calendario. Algunos meses tienen más de 4 semanas. El embarazo dura 280 días o cerca de 40 semanas. En realidad, un embarazo normal es cualquier embarazo que dure entre el principio de la 37 semana y el final de la 42 semana. Si tu bebé nace antes de la 37 semana, es considerado como prematuro. Si tu bebé nace despues de la 42 semana, es considerado postmaturo.

Special Instructions _____

_____

_____

_____

Phone number to call if you have questions: _____

Copyright © 2002 Lippincott Williams & Wilkins. Developed by MC Freda, EdD, RN, CHES, FAAN.

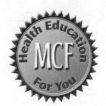

Woman's name: _____

Date: _____

Nurse's name: _____

The AFP Triple Test

What Is the AFP Test?

- The AFP Test is a special blood test for pregnant women that looks for the amount of AFP (alpha fetoprotein) in the woman's blood. At some hospitals, this test is called a "Double Test," a "Triple Test," or a "Quad Test" because the test can look for other chemicals at the same time. These chemicals are proteins made by the baby's body. They pass into the woman's blood through the afterbirth (placenta).

Why Is the AFP Test Done?

- The AFP Triple Test tells us if the baby is making too little, too much or just enough of these chemicals.
- Babies who make too much AFP <u>might</u> have a birth defect called neural tube defect (NTD). This means an opening in the spine or brain.
- Babies who make too little AFP and other chemicals <u>might</u> have Down syndrome, a genetic disease that includes mental retardation.
- High or low results <u>do not mean that there is something wrong with your baby</u>—only that you need further tests to see if something is wrong.

How Is the AFP Triple Test Done?

- It is a blood test, like other blood tests you have had. A small amount of blood is taken from your arm. The test can only be done between the 14th and 19th weeks of pregnancy. Your provider should explain the test to you before you decide to have it. You must agree to have the test done. No one can force you to do it.

What Happens After the AFP Triple Test Is Done?

- The doctors, nurses, or midwives will get the results of your AFP Triple Test and tell you the results. If the levels of AFP and the other chemicals are too high or too low, they might ask a genetic counselor to call you with the results and tell you about other tests that should be done. No other test will be done unless you give your permission.

Should You Have the AFP Test Done?

- Although most tests show that the baby is normal, some tests show problems. You should talk to your doctor, nurse, or midwife about what all this means and whether you want to have the test.

Remember that almost all AFP Triple Tests turn out to be normal. We are interested in helping to find out that <u>your baby</u> is healthy.

Ask your doctor, nurse, or midwife to explain anything you don't understand.

Flesch-Kincaid Reading Level: 5.14

Special Instructions _____

_____

Phone number to call if you have questions: _____

Copyright © 2002 Lippincott Williams & Wilkins. Developed by MC Freda, EdD, RN, CHES, FAAN.

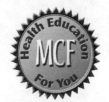

Woman's name: _____

Date: _____

Nurse's name: _____

LA PRUEBA TRIPLE DE LA AFP

¿Qué es la Prueba Triple de la AFP?

- La Prueba Triple de la AFP es una prueba especial de sangre para las mujeres embarazadas que examina la cantidad de AFP(Alfa Fetoproteina) y 2 otros químicos en la sangre de la mujer. El AFP y los otros 2 químicos son proteinas que su bebé produce. Estos pasan dentro de la sangre de la mujer a través de la placenta.

¿Porqué se hace la Prueba AFP?

- La Prueba AFP Triple nos indica si el bebé está produciendo muy poco, mucho o lo suficiente de estos químicos.
- Bebés que producen mucha AFP <u>pueden</u> tener un defecto de nacimiento llamado Defecto del Tubo Neural (DTN). Esto es una abertura en la espina dorsal ó el cerebro.
- Bebés que producen muy poco AFP y otros químicos <u>pueden</u> tener el Síndrome de Down, una enfermedad genética, la cual incluye el retrazo mental.
- Resultados bajos o altos <u>no quieren decir que haya algo malo con su bebé</u>—sólo que necesita más pruebas para ver si algo está mal.

¿Cómo Se Hace La Prueba Triple de la AFP?

- Es una prueba de sangre, como cualquier otra prueba de sangre que usted haya tenido. Una pequeña cantidad de sangre es tomada de su brazo. La prueba solamente se puede hacer entre la 14ta y 19na semana de su embarazo. Su proveedor de salud debe explicarle la prueba antes de que usted decida tenerla. Usted debe estar de acuerdo en hacerse la prueba. Nadie la puede forzar a tenerla.

¿Qué Es Lo Que Ocurre Después Que La Prueba Triple Se Haga?

- Los doctores, enfermeras, o parteras obtendrán los resultados de su Prueba Triple AFP y le dirán los resultados. Si los niveles del AFP y los otros químicos son muy altos o muy bajos, pueden pedirle a un/a consejero/a de génetica que la llame con los resultados y le diga que otras pruebas se deben hacer. Ninguna otra prueba se hará a menos que Usted dé su permiso.

¿Debe Hacerse La Prueba Triple de la AFP?

- A pesar de que la mayoría de las pruebas muestran que el bebé es normal, algunas pruebas podrían indicar que hay problemas. Debe hablar con su doctor, enfermera o partera sobre lo que esto significa, y si es que desea hacerse la prueba.

Acuérdese que casi todas las Pruebas Triples del AFP resultan normales. Estamos interesados en ayudarla a saber si es que <u>su bebé</u> está sano/a.

Pídale a su doctor, enfermera o partera que le explique cualquier cosa que no entienda.

Special Instructions _____

_____

Phone number to call if you have questions: _____

Copyright © 2002 Lippincott Williams & Wilkins. Developed by MC Freda, EdD, RN, CHES, FAAN.

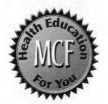

Woman's name: _____

Date: _____

Nurse's name: _____

Cigarette Smoking and Pregnancy

Do you smoke cigarettes?

If you are smoking and you are pregnant, you need to stop smoking right away. Cutting down is a good idea, but stopping is better. There is a lot of research that shows that smoking in pregnancy is very dangerous not only for you, but also for your baby.

Why do people keep smoking when it's bad for them?

Most women probably know that smoking cigarettes can give them cancer, or make asthma worse, or cause them to cough a lot. Most women who smoke continue to smoke because they are addicted to cigarettes. The nicotine in cigarettes is an addictive drug, and that makes it hard for some women to quit. But they must, for their own health and for their baby's health.

What are the effects of smoking on pregnancy?

There are thousands of poisonous chemicals in tobacco, and they go right to the baby. Those chemicals can cause the baby to be born too soon. They also cause low birth-weight, meaning that the baby does not gain enough weight during the pregnancy to be healthy when it is born.

How can you stop smoking?

There are special programs you can go to that will help you stop smoking. You should ask your doctor, nurse, or midwife if there are special smoking cessation programs at your hospital or birthing center. You can also call the American Lung Association at (212) 315-8700 or go to its Website at http://www.lungusa.com. Members of the association are experts at helping people to stop smoking, and they can advise you about how to do it and where you can find programs in your community.

Flesch-Kincaid Reading Level: 6.5

Special Instructions _____

_____

_____

_____

Phone number to call if you have questions: _____

Copyright © 2002 Lippincott Williams & Wilkins. Developed by MC Freda, EdD, RN, CHES, FAAN.

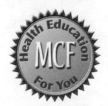

Woman's name: _____
Date: _____
Nurse's name: _____

Fumar Cigarrillo y el Embarazo

¿Fumas cigarillos?

Si fumas cigarrillos y estás embarazada, necesitas dejar de fumar de immediato. Recortar de fumar es muy buena idea, pero parar de fumar es mejor todavía. Hay muchos estudios que demuestran que el fumar durante el embarazo es muy peligroso, no solamente para tí, sino también para el bebé.

¿Porqué las personas siguen fumando sabiendo que es dañino para ellos?

Muchas mujeres probablemente saben que el fumar cigarrillos puede causar cáncer, o empeorar el asma, o causar mucha tós. Muchas mujeres que fuman, continuan haciéndolo porque son adictas al cigarrillo. La nicotina en el cigarrillo es una droga adictiva, ésto hace más difícil el poder dejar de fumar. Pero ellas deben de hacerlo, por su propia salud, y por la salud del bebé.

¿Cuáles son los efectos de fumar durante el embarazo?

Hay miles de químicos venenosos en el tabaco, y ellos pasan al bebé. Esos químicos causan que el bebé nazca antes de tiempo (prematuro). Tambien causa poco peso al nacer lo que significa que el bebé no aumenta de peso lo suficiente como para que sea saludable al nacer.

¿Cómo puedes parar de fumar?

Hay programas especiales donde puedes ir y te ayudaran a parar de fumar. Debes consultar con tu doctor, enfermera o comadrona, para saber si existen estos programas en tu hospital o en la maternidad. También puedes escribir a la Asociación Americana del Pulmón al (212)315-8700, o entrar a la página del internet http://www.lungusa.com. Hay personal expertos que ayudan a personas que tratan de dejar de fumar, ellos pueden aconcejarte como hacerlo, y donde puedes encontrar estos programas en tu comunidad.

Special Instructions _____

_____

_____

_____

Phone number to call if you have questions: _____

Copyright © 2002 Lippincott Williams & Wilkins. Developed by MC Freda, EdD, RN, CHES, FAAN.

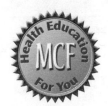

Woman's name: _____

Date: _____

Nurse's name: _____

The Problem of Partner Abuse

All women should be aware of the problem of partner abuse. The American College of Obstetricians and Gynecologists, the American College of Nurse Midwifery, and the major nursing organizations have all advised providers of care to give information to women about the problem of partner abuse. Because of this, we give you the following "abuse assessment," a simple 4-question survey. This survey is for your personal use only—you don't have to write anything on it. If you answer "yes" to any of the questions on the survey, please talk to your provider about it. He or she will help you to find help.

Assessment

1. Have you ever been emotionally or physically abused by your partner or someone important to you?
   Yes
   No

2. Within the last year, have you been hit, slapped, kicked, or otherwise physically hurt by someone?
   Yes
   No
   If yes, by whom?
   If yes, where on your body have you been hurt?

3. Within the last year, has anyone forced you to have sexual activities?
   Yes
   No
   If yes, who?
   If yes, how many times?

4. Are you afraid of your partner or anyone else?
   Yes
   No

Flesch-Kincaid Reading Level: 4.4

Special Instructions _____

_____

_____

_____

Phone number to call if you have questions: _____

Copyright © 2002 Lippincott Williams & Wilkins. Developed by MC Freda, EdD, RN, CHES, FAAN.

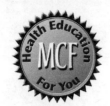

Woman's name: _____

Date: _____

Nurse's name: _____

Problema de Abuso de Pareja

Toda mujer debe estar alerta del problema de abuso de pareja. El Colegio Americano de Ginecólogos y Obstetras, el Colegio Americano de Enfermeras Parteras y las mayores organizaciones de enfermeras han recomendado a los proveedores de salud para dar información a las mujeres sobre el problema de abuso de pareja. Por esto le damos la siguiente "evaluación", unas 4 simples preguntas basadas en una investigación hecha en la Universidad de Johns Hopkins. Estas preguntas son para su uso personal solamente - no tienen que escribir nada. Si su respuesta es "sí" a cualquiera de las preguntas, por favor hable con su proveedor de salud al respecto. El ó ella le ayudará a buscar ayuda.

Cuestionario

1. ¿Ha sido usted alguna vez abusada física ó emocionalmente por su pareja o alguien importante para usted?
   Sí
   No

2. ¿Durante los últimos 12 meses ha sido usted golpeada, abofetada , pateada ó de otra forma maltratada físicamente por alguien?
   Sí
   No
   ¿Por quien?
   ¿En que parte de su cuerpo le han pegado?

3. ¿Durante los últimos 12 meses, alguien la ha forzado a tener sexo?
   Sí
   No
   ¿Quién?
   ¿Cuántas veces?

4. ¿Tiene miedo de su pareja u otra persona?
   Sí
   No

Special Instructions _____

_____

_____

_____

Phone number to call if you have questions: _____

Copyright © 2002 Lippincott Williams & Wilkins. Developed by MC Freda, EdD, RN, CHES, FAAN.

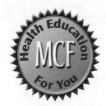

Woman's name: _____

Date: _____

Nurse's name: _____

Danger Assessment

Some women who are in violent relationships are in danger of being killed. We cannot predict what will happen in your case, but we would like you to be aware of the danger of homicide in situations of severe battering. You need to see how many of the risk factors apply to your situation. (The "he" in the question refers to your husband, partner, ex-husband, ex-partner or whoever is currently physically hurting you).

Please check YES or NO for each question below.

YES	NO	
____	____	1. Has the physical violence increased in frequency over the past year?
____	____	2. Has the physical violence increased in severity over the past year and/or has a weapon or threat with weapon been used?
____	____	3. Does he ever try to choke you?
____	____	4. Is there a gun in the house?
____	____	5. Has he ever forced you into sex when you did not wish to do so?
____	____	6. Does he use drugs? By drugs we mean uppers or amphetamines, speed, angel dust, cocaine, crack, street drugs, heroin, or mixtures.
____	____	7. Does he threaten to kill you and/or do you believe he is capable of killing you?
____	____	8. Is he drunk every day or almost every day?
____	____	9. Does he control most/all of your daily activities? For instance, does he tell you who you can be friends with, how much money you can take with you shopping, or when you can take the car? (If he tries, but you do not let him, check here____.)
____	____	10. Have you ever been beaten by him while you were pregnant? (If never pregnant by him, check here____.)
____	____	11. Is he violently and constantly jealous of you? (For instance, does he say, "If I can't have you, no one can?")
____	____	12. Have you ever threatened or tried to commit suicide?
____	____	13. Has he ever threatened or tried to commit suicide?
____	____	14. Is he violent outside of the home?
____	____	TOTAL YES ANSWERS

Thank you. Please complete this form and then show it to your nurse, doctor, midwife, advocate, or counselor. Talk to them about what the danger assessment means in terms of your situation.

Developed by J Campbell, PhD, RN

Special Instructions _____

_____

_____

Phone number to call if you have questions: _____

Copyright © 2002 Lippincott Williams & Wilkins. Developed by MC Freda, EdD, RN, CHES, FAAN.

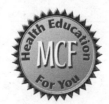

Woman's name: _____

Date: _____

Nurse's name: _____

Evaluación de Peligro

Algunas mujeres que estan en relaciones violentas corren peligro de ser asesinadas. No podemos predecir que sucederá en su caso, pero me gustaría advertirle del peligro de homicidio en situaciones de abuso severo y que usted se dé cuenta de cuantos factores de riesgo se aplican en su situación. (En las siguientes preguntas cuando hablamos de "él" nos estamos refiriendo a su marido, compañero, ex-marido, ex compañero o quienquiera que la esté actualmente dañando físicamente.)

Por favor marque SI o NO a cada una de las preguntas que siguen a continuación.

SI	NO	
_____	_____	1. ¿Ha aumentado su compañero la violencia física durante el año pasado?
_____	_____	2. ¿Ha aumentado la severidad de violencia física por su compañero durante el año pasado y/o ha habido el uso de un arma, o has sido amenazada con un arma?
_____	_____	3. ¿Ha tratado él de asfixiarla?
_____	_____	4. ¿Hay algún arma de fuego en su casa?
_____	_____	5. ¿La ha forzado él a tener relaciones sexuales en contra de su voluntad?
_____	_____	6. ¿Usa él drogas? Por drogas me refiero a exitantes o anfetaminas, "speed," polvo de ángel, cocaína, crack, drogas de la calle, heroína, o mezclas.
_____	_____	7. ¿La amenaza él con matarla o cree usted que él es capaz de matarla?
_____	_____	8. ¿Se emborracha él todos los días o casi todos los días? (Refiérase a la cantidad de alcohol.)
_____	_____	9. ¿Controla él la mayoría de sus actividades diarias? Por ejemplo, ¿le dice él quienes pueden ser sus amistades, o cuanto dinero puede llevar cuando va de compras, o cuando puede usar el coche? (Si él trata, pero usted no lo deja, marque aquí___.)
_____	_____	10. ¿Ha sido usted golpeada cuando estaba embarazada? (Si no ha estado embarazada de él, marque aquí___.)
_____	_____	11. ¿Es él violento, o constantemente celoso de usted? Por ejemplo le dice él: "Si no eres mía no vas a serlo de nadie."
_____	_____	12. ¿Ha usted amenazado o tratado de suicidarse?
_____	_____	13. ¿Ha tratado o amenazado él de suicidarse?
_____	_____	14. ¿Es él violento fuera de la casa?
_____	_____	TOTAL DE RESPUESTAS SI

Gracias. Por favor hable con su enfermera, su enfermera-comadrona certificada, su doctor, asesor legal, o consejero sobre lo que la evaluación de peligro significa en su caso.

De J Campbell, PhD, RN

Special Instructions _____

_____

Phone number to call if you have questions: _____

Copyright © 2002 Lippincott Williams & Wilkins. Developed by MC Freda, EdD, RN, CHES, FAAN.

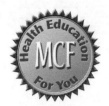

MCF
Health Education
For You

Woman's name: _____

Date: _____

Nurse's name: _____

Nutritional Guidelines in Pregnancy

What is a good diet in pregnancy? First of all, <u>don't diet</u>!! If you starve yourself, you also starve your baby, so during your pregnancy eat <u>good, nutritious food</u>, and you will lose your pregnancy weight gain after your baby is born. The U.S. Department of Agriculture says that a good nutritious diet in pregnancy includes these things:

Food Category:	Examples of one serving:
Breads, Cereals, Whole Grains 6-11 servings daily	1 slice bread, ½ hamburger bun or English muffin, 3-4 small or 2 large crackers, 1/2 cup cooked pasta or rice
Fruits 2-4 servings daily	¾ cup juice, 1 medium apple or banana
Vegetables 3-5 servings daily	½ cup cooked or chopped raw vegetables 1 cup leafy raw vegetables
Meat, Poultry, Fish 6-7 ounces daily	1 egg, ½ cup cooked beans, 2 tablespoons peanut butter
Milk, Cheese, Yogurt 4 servings daily	1 cup milk, 8 ounces yogurt, 1½ ounces cheese

How much weight do women usually gain during pregnancy? A weight gain of 28 pounds is normal, but you could gain 22 to 35 pounds. If you're underweight, you might gain more, and if you're overweight you might gain less, but everyone needs to gain some weight during pregnancy.

Calories. Most women need about 300 added calories each day when pregnant. This is about 2½ cups of low-fat milk, 1 cup of ice cream, a bagel with cream cheese, or a tuna fish sandwich.

Protein. Pregnant women need extra protein, like that in 1¼ cups of milk or 1½ ounces of red meat.

Calcium. Twice as much calcium is needed in pregnancy. Eat green leafy vegetables, orange juice, milk, yogurt, and cheese.

Iron. You need extra iron: fish, poultry, whole grain breads and cereals, green leafy vegetables, legumes, dried fruits, eggs, liver, and red meat.

Caffeine. Some new studies say that caffeine can increase the risk of miscarriage. Avoiding caffeine in pregnancy is a probably a good idea.

Food Cravings. No one really knows why these happen, but they are probably not the result of food deficiencies. There is no reason to avoid foods you crave unless they are high in fat or calorie content and could therefore cause large weight gain.

Flesch-Kincaid Reading Level:6.4

Special Instructions _____

Phone number to call if you have questions: _____

Copyright © 2002 Lippincott Williams & Wilkins. Developed by MC Freda, EdD, RN, CHES, FAAN.

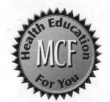

Woman's name: _____

Date: _____

Nurse's name: _____

Guías Nutricionales para el Embarazo

¿Qué es una buena dieta para el embarazo? Primero que nada, ¡No Haga Dieta! si usted se muere de hambre, también matará de hambre a su bebé, así que durante su embarazo aliméntese bien, alimentos nutritivos y el peso que usted ganó durante el embarazo lo perderá después que nazca el bebé. El Departamento de Agricultura de los Estados Unidos dice que una buena dieta nutritiva incluye lo siguiente:

Categoría de Comida:	Ejemplos de una porción
Panes, Cereales, Granos Enteros De 6 a 11 porciones diarias	Una tajada de pan, ½ pan de hamburguesa o un English Muffin ,de 3 a 4 galletas pequeñas ó 2 grandes, ½ taza de pasta cocida, o arroz
Frutas De 2 a 4 porciones diarias	¾ de taza de jugo, 1 manzana o banana mediano
Vegetales De 3 a 5 porciones diarias	½ taza de vegetales cocidos o crudos cortados en trozos
Carne, Aves de Corral, Pescado De 6 a 7 onzas diarias	Un huevo, ½ taza de frijoles cocidos, Dos cucharadas de mantequilla de maní
Leche, Queso, Yogur 4 porciones diarias	1 taza de leche, ocho onzas de yogur 1½ onzas de queso

¿Generalmente cuánto peso aumentan las mujeres durante el embarazo? Un aumento de 28 libras es normal, sin embargo usted puede aumentar de veinte y dos a treinta y cinco libras, si usted está bajo en peso, puede aumentar más y si usted tiene sobre peso, puede aumentar menos, pero todas necesitan aumentar algo de peso durante sus embarazos.

Calorías. La mayoría de las mujeres, mientras estan embarazadas necesitan cada día aumentar alrededor de 300 calorías. Esto es como dos tazas y media de leche baja en grasa, una taza de helado, un bagel con crema de queso o un sandwich de atún

Proteínas. Las mujeres embarazadas necesitan proteína extra como la que se encuentra en una taza y media de leche o en una onza y media de carne roja.

Calcio. Durante el embarazo se necesita dos veces más calcio. Consuma vegetales con hojas verdes, jugo de naranja, leche, yogur y quesos.

Hierro. Usted necesita hierro extra: pescado,aves de corral, panes con granos enteros y cereals, vegetales con hojas verdes, legumbres, frutas secas, huevos, hígado y carnes rojas.

Cafeína. Algunos estudios nuevos muestran de que la cafeína puede aumentar el riesgo de abortar. El evitar la cafeína durante el embarazo es probablemente una buena idea.

Antojos de Comida. En realidad nadie sabe porqué sucede ésto, pero probablemente no son el producto de deficiencias de alimentos. No existe ninguna razón para evitar los alimentos que se le antojan a menos de que contengan mucha grasa o calorías y como consecuencia puedan causar mucho aumento de peso.

Special Instructions _____

_____

Phone number to call if you have questions: _____

Copyright © 2002 Lippincott Williams & Wilkins. Developed by MC Freda, EdD, RN, CHES, FAAN.

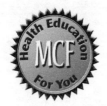

Woman's name: _____

Date: _____

Nurse's name: _____

Tests in Pregnancy

There are many laboratory tests that will be done during your pregnancy to see if you and your baby are healthy. Some tests can only be done at certain times in pregnancy, so it's very important to have the tests done when they are ordered.

These Tests Might Be Done at Your First Prenatal Visit

Blood tests

Complete Blood Count (CBC) or Hemoglobin and Hematocrit—to see if you are anemic

Syphilis—required by law to be sure you are not infected

Rubella—to see if you have had German measles or need the vaccine after the birth

Blood type and Rh positive. If you are Rh negative, you need further testing and treatment

Hepatitis—to find out if you have been infected with this virus

Alpha fetoprotein (also called "Double Screen,""Triple Screen," or "Quad Test")—to see if further testing is necessary to find spina bifida or Down syndrome

Skin test

Tuberculosis (PPD)—a skin test to see if you have been exposed to tuberculosis

Urine test

Urine culture—to check for any infection

Other tests

PAP Test—to check for cervical disease

Pregnancy test—either blood or urine

These Tests Might Be Done at Each Visit, Depending on Your Provider

Urine "Dipstick"—to check for glucose and protein

Your weight and blood pressure

The "Fundal Height"—measuring the size of your uterus from the outside

Fetal heart rate—listening to the baby's heart (after 10 weeks of pregnancy)

Additional or Optional Tests

Genetic testing—offered to families with special risks

HIV blood test—now recommended by many states to be done for every pregnant woman. If the test is positive for the HIV virus, medicines can be given to the woman to help prevent transmitting the virus to the baby

Glucose challenge test—a blood test for diabetes in pregnancy performed between 26 and 28 weeks of pregnancy.

Cultures of your cervix for: chlamydia, gonorrhea, herpes, and group B strep—if any of these things are present, they can possibly cause problems for the baby and require treatment

Ultrasound (also called sonogram)—might be done to check on the baby's growth or to look for problems in the baby

Flesch-Kincaid Reading Level: 6.8

Special Instructions _____

Phone number to call if you have questions: _____

Copyright © 2002 Lippincott Williams & Wilkins. Developed by MC Freda, EdD, RN, CHES, FAAN.

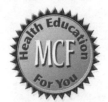

Woman's name: _____

Date: _____

Nurse's name: _____

Exámenes durante el Embarazo

Existen muchos exámenes de laboratorio que se le harán durante su embarazo para ver si usted y su bebé estan saludables. Algunos exámenes son hechos solamente en ciertas etapas del embarazo, así que es muy importante que se haga éstas pruebas cuando sean ordenadas por su proveedor.

Estos exámenes pueden hacerse durante la primera visita prenatal:

Exámenes de sangre:

Exámen completo de sangre (CBC) o Hemoglobina y Hematocritos-detecta si usted está anémica
Sífilis-requerido por la ley para asegurarse que no esté infectada.
Rubeola-para detectar si ha tenido el sarampión, o necesita la vacuna después del parto
Tipo de Sangre y RH positivo-Si eres RH negativo, necesitarás otras pruebas y tratamiento.
Hepatitis-para saber si has estado infectada por el virus.
Alfa Fetoproteína-para determinar si es necesario otras pruebas para la detección de Espina Bífida o el Síndrome de Down.

Pruebas de la piel:

Tuberculosis(PPD)-una prueba en la piel para detectar si has estado expuesta al virus de la tuberculosis

Exámen de orina-

para chequear cualquier infección

Otras pruebas:

Exámen del Papnicolaou (PAP)- para chequear enfermedades de la cervix
Exámen de embarazo-puede ser de orina o de sangre.

Estos exámenes pueden hacerse en cada visita, dependiendo de su proveedor:

Exámen de orina -usando una tira reactiva para chequear la glucosa y proteína.
Peso y Presión arterial
Medida del útero- medida que se hace desde afuera.
Frecuencia cardíaca del feto- escucha el corazón del bebé (después de la 10ma semana de embarazo)

Exámenes adicionales u opcionales:

Pruebas genéticas-para aquellas personas con problemas especiales.
Prueba del VIH- es recomendado que se le haga a todas las mujeres embarazadas, aprobado en muchos estados de la nación. Si el resultado es positivo, se le administraran medicamentos para prevenir la transmición del virus al bebé.
Exámen de la glucosa-un exámen de sangre para detectar la diabetes en el embarazo, se hace entre la 26-28 semanas de embarazo.
Muestras del cervix- para detectar clamidia, gonorrea, herpes o Strep del grupo B- si cualquiera de estas enfermedades están presentes, pueden causar problemas para el bebé y necesitara tratamiento.
Ultrasonido (tambien conocido como Sonograma)- es efectuado para chequear el desarollo del bebé, o para detectar algun problema con el bebé.

Special Instructions _____

Phone number to call if you have questions: _____

Copyright © 2002 Lippincott Williams & Wilkins. Developed by MC Freda, EdD, RN, CHES, FAAN.

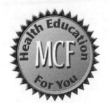

Woman's name: _____

Date: _____

Nurse's name: _____

Fetal Movement Counting

Your doctor, nurse, or midwife might tell you to count your baby's movements every day. This is done (usually toward the end of pregnancy) to be sure that your baby is healthy, because a baby who moves a lot is usually a healthy baby. Not all babies move around the same amount. So while your friend's baby might move all day and all night, you might have a quieter baby who likes to sleep. That's why you need to pay attention to your own baby's movements and keep track of when he or she is the most active. There are several different ways of checking for your baby's movements. Your provider might tell you to count after meals, or first thing in the morning, or around bedtime. No matter when you start counting, here are the most important things for you do:

- You probably know your baby's quiet times and his or her awake times. Choose a time when your baby is usually awake and moving. Sit down or lie down in a quiet place. Do nothing but pay attention to your baby's movements. Don't have conversations with anyone, because you'll easily lose count!

- Mark down on a paper what time you started paying attention. Make a mark each time you feel the baby move.

- Unless the baby is sleeping, it will usually move at least 4 times in an hour. If your baby does not move at least 3 times during the hour you choose to count, then keep counting until you get to 4 movements. If your baby does not move at least 4 times in several hours, you need to call your doctor, nurse, or midwife right away. He or she will want to know about this and perhaps do some tests to see how the baby is.

Flesch-Kincaid Reading Level: 5.8

Special Instructions _____

_____

_____

_____

_____

_____

_____

Phone number to call if you have questions: _____

Copyright © 2002 Lippincott Williams & Wilkins. Developed by MC Freda, EdD, RN, CHES, FAAN.

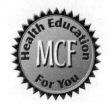

Woman's name: _____

Date: _____

Nurse's name: _____

Contando el Movimiento Fetal

Tu doctor, enfermera ó comadrona podrían decirte que cuentes los movimientos del bebé diariamente. Esto es hecho (por lo general al final del embarazo) para asegurarse que el bebé esté saludable, porque un bebé que se mueve mucho, por lo general indica que está saludable. No todos los bebés se mueven en la misma cantidad. Mientras que el bebé de tu amiga se mueve todo el día y la noche, tú tienes en cambio un bebé más tranquilo que le gusta dormir. Por eso es que tienes que prestar atención a los movimientos del bebé, y llevar un record de cuando el ó la bebé está más activo(a). Hay diferentes formas de chequear los movimientos del bebé. Tu doctor puede decirte que cuentes después de las comidas, o temprano en la mañana ó al acostarse. No importa cuando comienzes a hacerlo, lo importante es qué debes hacer:

• Probablemente sepas cuando son los momentos menos activos y cuando está despierto(a). Escoge el momento cuando el bebé esté despierto(a) y activo. Siéntate o acuéstate en un sitio tranquilo. No hagas nada, solamente presta atención a los movimientos de tu bebé. No converses con nadie, por lo que podrías perder la cuenta!!

• Escribe en un papel la hora cuando empezastes a prestar atención. Haz una marca cada vez que el bebé se mueva.

• A menos que el bebé esté dormido, éste(a) se mueve por lo menos 4 veces en una hora. Si tu bebé no se mueve al menos 3 veces durante la hora que escogistes para contar, entonces sigue contando hasta que obtengas 4 movimientos. Si tu bebé no se mueve al menos 4 veces en varias horas, necesitarás llamar de immediato a tu doctor, enfermera o comadrona. Ellos necesitarán saber sobre esto y quizás tendrían que hacerte unas pruebas para saber como está el bebé.

Special Instructions _____

_____

_____

_____

_____

_____

Phone number to call if you have questions: _____

Copyright © 2002 Lippincott Williams & Wilkins. Developed by MC Freda, EdD, RN, CHES, FAAN.

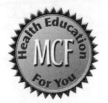

Woman's name: _____

Date: _____

Nurse's name: _____

Sexually Transmitted Diseases

You should understand more about sexually transmitted diseases (STDs) and some of the STD tests you will be having during pregnancy. Most women who have only one sexual partner don't think about being at risk for STDs. You might not have any symptoms, but you still need to be tested for STDs during pregnancy, because if you have one, the baby can get it, and can become very sick. If you think you have an STD, be sure to tell your doctor, nurse, or midwife.

Chlamydia, Gonorrhea, and PID

Chlamydia ("klah-mid-ee-ah") and gonorrhea ("gone-or-ee-ah") infections are the most common STDs in the United States today. Chlamydia and gonorrhea infections can cause PID (pelvic inflammatory disease), a severe infection that spreads from the vagina and cervix to the uterus, fallopian tubes, and ovaries. If this happens, you could become infertile. Chlamydia and gonorrhea **can be treated and can be cured with medicine.** Chlamydia and gonorrhea can infect the fetus as it passes through the vagina during the birth, causing eye infections, lung infections, and other complications. A newborn's eyes are very sensitive, and blindness may result. To help prevent this, the eyes of all newborns are treated at birth. This is done for every baby whether or not the mother has a history of gonorrhea.

Herpes Simplex Virus

Genital herpes ("her-pees") is an infection caused by herpes simplex virus. It produces sores and blisters on or around the sex organs and is transmitted during sex through direct contact with a person who has active sores. Some people have only one outbreak in their lives, while others have many. If a pregnant woman has herpes simplex, the baby can become infected during birth. As a result the baby may suffer some severe effects. If you have ever had genital herpes, or had sexual contact with someone who has, tell your provider. If there are signs of active infection when you are in labor, your provider may plan for a cesarean birth, which can reduce the chance that the baby will come into contact with the virus in the vagina.

Human Papillomavirus

Human papillomavirus (HPV) ("pap-ill-oma") causes genital warts. Warts in the genital area are easily passed from person to person during vaginal, oral, and anal sex. If you think you have genital warts, let your doctor know. Tests need to be done to find out if the infection has spread.

Syphilis

Syphilis ("sif-ah-liss") is a dangerous STD, and if untreated can spread throughout the body and cause lifelong illness. Syphilis can be passed from a pregnant women's bloodstream to her fetus, sometimes causing miscarriage or stillbirth. If the infant lives, he or she may be born with syphilis. **Syphilis can be treated**, and therefore you will be tested for it.

HIV

HIV is an STD. There is a separate handout about HIV. Please read it.

Be sure to talk to your doctor, nurse, or midwife about STDs and their treatment.

Flesch-Kincaid Reading Level: 8.6

Special Instructions _____

Phone number to call if you have questions: _____

Copyright © 2002 Lippincott Williams & Wilkins. Developed by MC Freda, EdD, RN, CHES, FAAN.

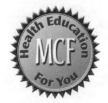

Woman's name: _____

Date: _____

Nurse's name: _____

Enfermedades Transmitidas Sexualmente

Usted debería de entender más sobre las enfermedades transmitidas sexualmente(STD) y sobre algunas de las pruebas del STD a las que será sometida durante su embarazo. La mayoría de las mujeres que solamente tienen una pareja sexual, no piensan que puedan estar expuestas a contraer enfermedades transmitidas sexualmente. Quizás no muestre ningún síntoma. Más sin embargo todavía necesita hacerse las pruebas del STD durante su embarazo, porque si usted está infectada, su bebé podría contraer la enfermedad y enfermarse severamente. Si usted cree de que tiene una enfermedad transmitida sexualmente asegúrese de comunicárselo a su doctor, enfermera ó comadrona.

Clamidia, Gonorrea y Enfermedad Inflamatoria de la Pelvis

Las infecciones de clamidia y gonorrea son las enfermedades sexuales más comunes en los Estados Unidos hoy en día. Las infeccins de clamidia y gonorrea pueden causar enfermedad inflamatoria de la pelvis (PID), es una infección muy severa que se riega desde la vagina y cervix hasta el útero, tubos de fallopio y ovarios. Si ésto sucede, usted podría quedar infértil. La clamidia y gonorrea pueden ser **tratada y pueden ser curadas con medicinas**. Estas pueden infectar el feto , cuando la infección pasa a través de la vagina durante el parto, causando infecciones de los ojos, infección del pulmón y otras complicaciones. Los ojos de un bebé recién nacido son muy sensitivos, y la ceguera podría ocurrir. Para prevenir ésto, los ojos de un recién nacido son tratados al nacimiento. Esto es hecho por cada bebé sin importar sin la madre tiene un historial de gonorrea o no.

Herpes Simple

Herpes genital es una infección causada por el virus del herpes simple. Produce úlceras y ampollas sobre o alrededor de los órganos sexuales. Es transmitida durante el acto sexual con una persona que tenga úlceras activas. Algunas personas solo sufren un episodio en su vida, mientras que otras pueden experimentar muchas más. Si una persona embarazada tiene herpes simple, el bebé puede infectarse durante el nacimiento. Como resultado el bebé podría sufrir graves consecuencias. Si usted alguna vez ha sufrido de herpes genital, o ha tenido contacto con una persona que la tenga, consulte de immediato con su doctor. Si hay señales de infección activa durante el parto, su doctor decidirá por un parto por cesárea, el cual reduce el riesgo de que su bebé se ponga en contacto con el virus en la vagina.

Human papillovirus

Papillomas virus causan verrugas genitales. Estas verrugas son transmitidas muy fácilmente de persona a persona durante el sexo anal, vaginal y oral. Si usted cree que tiene verrugas genitales, hable con su doctor. Tendrá que hacerse unos exámenes para detectar si el virus se ha esparcido.

Sífilis

Sífilis es una de las enfermedades transmitida sexualmente de más peligro, si se deja sin tratamiento se puede esparcer por todo el cuerpo y puede causar muchas enfermedades crónicas. Esta enfermedad se transmite al feto a través del sistema circulatorio de la madre, alguna veces causando el aborto o produciendo el parto de un bebé muerto. Si el infante sobrevive, puede que éste(a) nazca con sífiles. **Sífiles puede ser tratado,** por lo tanto hágase un exámen.

VIH

VIH es una enfermedad transmitida sexualmente. Hay un folleto separado sobre el VIH. Por favor léalo.

Asegúrese de hablar con su doctor, enfermera o comadrona sobre las enfermedades transmitidas sexualmente y su tratamiento.

Special Instructions _____

Phone number to call if you have questions: _____

Copyright © 2002 Lippincott Williams & Wilkins. Developed by MC Freda, EdD, RN, CHES, FAAN.

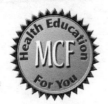

Woman's name: _____

Date: _____

Nurse's name: _____

What You Need to Know About Having the HIV Test in Pregnancy

1. There are some behaviors that can put you at higher risk of developing HIV:
   Having sex with someone who has HIV
   Having anal sex
   Using IV drugs, having sex with an IV drug user, or sharing needles
2. The purpose of the HIV blood test is to tell if your blood has the HIV antibodies. It does not tell if you have active AIDS.
3. Your health care provider will tell you the results of your test. If the HIV test is "Positive" it means you have HIV antibodies in your blood, and we will refer you for treatment.
4. If you have HIV, it is good to know right away because you can get medical treatment. Taking medication for this during pregnancy could keep your baby from getting HIV.
5. No one can force you to have the test. It is voluntary.
6. If you want the test to be anonymous (without your name used), you can usually do that at the health department.
7. If your test is positive for HIV, some states require that the names of your known sexual contacts be reported. This is done to help stop the spread of the disease. You should ask if your state requires this. If so, your known sexual contacts will be notified that they have been exposed to HIV, but your name will not be disclosed. Some states allow you to notify your sexual contacts instead of the state doing it. Be sure to ask about this.
8. If you are concerned about the possibility of physical abuse when telling a sexual contact about a positive HIV test, tell us so we can get help for you.
9. Legal protection is available to you if anyone discriminates against you because of being HIV positive.

Based on NYS Public Health Law 2781

Flesch-Kincaid Reading Level: 6.2

Special Instructions _____

_____

_____

_____

_____

Phone number to call if you have questions: _____

Copyright © 2002 Lippincott Williams & Wilkins. Developed by MC Freda, EdD, RN, CHES, FAAN.

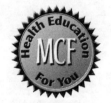

Lo que necesita saber sobre la prueba del VIH en el embarazo

1. Hay comportamientos que la pueden poner a un mayor riesgo de desarrollar el VIH:
   Al tener relaciones sexuales con alguien que tenga el VIH
   Al tener sexo anal
   Al usar drogas IV, al tener relaciones sexuales con alguien que use drogas IV, o que comparta agujas

2. El propósito de la prueba de sangre VIH es decirle si su sangre tiene los anticuerpos del VIH. No indica si tiene el SIDA activo.

3. Su proveedor de salud le dirá los resultados de su prueba. Si la prueba VIH es "Positiva" significa que su sangre tiene anticuerpos VIH, y le haremos un referido para su tratamiento.

4. Si tiene el VIH, es bueno saber de inmediato porque puede obtener tratamiento médico. Tomar medicamentos para esto durante su embarazo la puede ayudar a que su bebé no adquiera el VIH.

5. Nadie la puede forzar que se haga la prueba. Es voluntaria.

6. Si quiere que la prueba sea anónima (sin que su nombre sea usado), puede hacerlo en el Departamento de Salud.

7. Si su prueba es positiva para el VIH, algunos estados requieren que los nombres de su conocidos contactos sexuales sean reportados. Esto es hecho para ayudar a parar la propagación de la enfermedad. Debe preguntar si su estado requiere esto. Si este es el caso, sus contactos sexuales conocidos seran notificados que han sido expuestos al VIH, pero su nombre no será revelado.

8. Si está preocupada acerca de la posibilidad de abuso físico al comunicar a un contacto sexual de una prueba del VIH positivo, avísenos para que podamos conseguirle ayuda.

9. Protección legal es disponible para usted si alguna persona discrimina contra usted por ser VIH positiva.

Basado en la Ley de Salud NYS 2781

Special Instructions _____

_____

_____

_____

_____

Phone number to call if you have questions: _____

Copyright © 2002 Lippincott Williams & Wilkins. Developed by MC Freda, EdD, RN, CHES, FAAN.

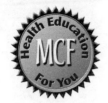

Woman's name: _____

Date: _____

Nurse's name: _____

Warning Signs in Pregnancy

There are some things that can happen in pregnancy that mean you need to see the doctor, nurse, or midwife right away. If any of these things happen to you, call your provider right away:

- **Bleeding from your vagina**

- **Severe pain, cramps, or abdominal pressure that does not go away**

- **Low dull backache**

- **Fainting or dizziness**

- **Severe headache or a headache that doesn't go away**

- **Sudden swelling in your hands, face, feet, or ankles**

- **Rapid weight gain**

- **Blurred vision or spots before your eyes**

- **Pain or burning when you urinate**

- **Chills or fever**

- **Severe nausea or vomiting**

- **A rash or unusual sores on your body**

- **Stopping or slowing down of the baby's movements**

- **Discharge from your vagina that is bloody, greenish, yellow, bad smelling, burning, or itchy**

Flesch-Kincaid Reading Level: 4.2

Special Instructions _____

_____

_____

_____

_____

Phone number to call if you have questions: _____

Copyright © 2002 Lippincott Williams & Wilkins. Developed by MC Freda, EdD, RN, CHES, FAAN.

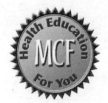

Woman's name: _____

Date: _____

Nurse's name: _____

Síntomas Peligrosos En El Embarazo

Cosas que pueden pasar en el embarazo que indican que usted necesita ver al doctor, enfermera o partera inmediatamente. Si cualquiera de estas cosas le sucede a usted, llame a su proveedor de salud de inmediato:

- **Sangrado de la vagina**
- **Severo dolor, calambres o presión abdominal que no se alivia**
- **Dolor en el área baja de la espalda**
- **Mareo ó desmayo**
- **Severo dolor de cabeza o dolor de cabeza que no se alivia**
- **Repentina hinchazón en sus manos, cara, pies o tobillos**
- **Aumento rápido de peso**
- **Visión borrosa o visión de manchas en frente de sus ojos**
- **Dolor o ardor al orinar**
- **Fiebre o escalofrío**
- **Severa nausea o vomito**
- **Una mancha o enrojecimiento inusual de la piel**
- **Que disminuyan o se paren los movimientos del bebé**
- **Flujo vaginal con mal olor, que arda o pique, de color verdoso, amarillento o sangriento.**

Special Instructions _____

_____

_____

_____

_____

_____

_____

Phone number to call if you have questions: _____

Copyright © 2002 Lippincott Williams & Wilkins. Developed by MC Freda, EdD, RN, CHES, FAAN.

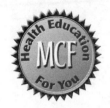

Woman's name: _____

Date: _____

Nurse's name: _____

Did You Know That Preterm Birth Can Be Dangerous to Your Baby's Health?

Preterm birth is any birth that happens before the thirty-seventh week of pregnancy. Pregnancy should last about 40 weeks. Babies born before 37 weeks may have many health problems and may need to stay in the hospital for extra days or weeks. The earlier your baby is born, the more health problems he or she may have. If preterm labor is recognized in time, it might be possible to stop the labor or to give you medicines that can help the baby's lungs to work better if he or she is born early. The most important thing that a pregnant woman can do to help prevent premature labor is to understand the symptoms of preterm labor and to take action if the symptoms occur. Watch for these signs, and if any of them happen to you, follow the instructions below:

Warning Signs of Preterm Labor

Cramps, like during your period (constant or comes and goes)
Low, dull backache (constant or comes and goes)
Pelvic pressure (feels like the baby is pushing down)
Abdominal cramps (with or without diarrhea)
Increased or changed vaginal discharge (mucousy or watery)
Uterine contractions, 10 minutes apart or closer, which may be painless (this might feel like the baby is "balling up" inside you; your uterus will feel hard and then soft)

What to Do If You Have Preterm Labor Symptoms

If you have **ANY** of the warning signs (you don't need to have them all) then you should stop what you are doing and:

- Lie down on your left side for 1 hour, and drink 2 to 3 glasses of water or juice.
- If the symptoms go away, you can go back to light activity, but not what you were doing when the symptoms began.
- If the symptoms get worse, call your doctor, nurse, or midwife or go right to the hospital.
- If the symptoms come back after that hour, call or go right to the hospital.

If you have any of these symptoms and they don't go away, waiting for hours before you are examined by a doctor or midwife *is not a good idea.* **You could be in preterm labor. If preterm labor is discovered early enough it may be stopped or medicines may be given to you to help the baby breathe better if he or she is born prematurely.**

Flesch-Kincaid Reading Level: 7.0

Special Instructions _____

Phone number to call if you have questions: _____

Copyright © 2002 Lippincott Williams & Wilkins. Developed by MC Freda, EdD, RN, CHES, FAAN.

MCF Health Education For You

¿Sabe Usted que un Parto Prematuro Puede Ser Peligroso para la Salud del Bebé?

Un parto prematuro es cualquier parto que ocurre antes de la 37va semana de gestación. Un embarazo debería de durar 40 semanas. Los bebés nacidos antes de la semana 37 de gestación pueden contraer muchas problemas de salud y pueda que necesiten quedarse en el hospital unos días extras e incluso semanas. Cuanto más temprano nazca el bebé, más problemas de salud el ó ella tendrá. Si se detecta a tiempo un parto prematuro, es posible detener el parto, o administrarles medicinas las cuales ayudan a que los pulmones del bebé trabajen más eficientemente si éste(a) naciera prematuramente. La cosa más importante que una mujer embarazada debe hacer para ayudar a prevenir un parto prematuro es tomar pronta acción si se presentara cualquiera de éstos síntomas. Observa estas señales y si cualquiera de ellas te suceden, sigue estas instrucciones:

Señales de advertencia de un parto prematuro

Calambres, como durante tu menstruación (constantes o que van y vienen)
Dolor en la parte baja de la espalda (constantes o que van y vienen)
Presión en la pelvis (se siente como si el bebé está empujando hacia abajo)
Calambres abdominales (con o sin diarrea)
Cambio ó incremento en el flujo vaginal (mucosidad o aguado)
Contracciones uterinas, 10 minutos aparte o menos, las cuales pueden ser sin dolor (se siente como si el bebé está dando "vueltas" dentro de tí; tu útero se sentirá rígido y luego blando)

Que hacer si tienes algunos de estos síntomas

Si experimentas **algunos** de estas señales de advertencia (no necesitas sentir todos estos síntomas a la vez) para todo lo que estabas haciendo y:

- Acuéstate en el lado izquierdo por una hora, y toma 2-3 vasos de agua o jugo.
- Si los síntomas se alivian, puedes hacer actividad ligera, pero no lo que estabas haciendo cuando se presentaron los síntomas.
- Si los síntomas empeoran, llama a tu doctor, enfermera ó comadrona ó ve directamente al hospital.
- Si los síntomas regresan después de una hora, llama o ve directamente al hospital.

   Si sientes algunos de estos síntomas y no se alivian, no dejes pasar varias horas sin antes llamar a tu doctor, NO ES UNA BUENA IDEA. **Podrías estar experimentando un parto prematuro. Si ésto es descubierto a tiempo, puede ser detenido ó se le administrarían medicinas para ayudar a que el bebé respire mejor si éste(a) llegara a nacer prematuramente.**

Special Instructions _____

_____

Phone number to call if you have questions: _____

Copyright © 2002 Lippincott Williams & Wilkins. Developed by MC Freda, EdD, RN, CHES, FAAN.

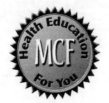

Woman's name: _____
Date: _____
Nurse's name: _____

What is Preeclampsia?

You might not have ever heard this word. Preeclampsia (pronounced "pree-ee-clamp-see-ah") is a disease that only happens in pregnancy. People used to call this "toxemia." About 6 in every 100 pregnant women develop preeclampsia, so you should know what it is, what the symptoms are, and when to call your provider if any of the symptoms happen to you.

Preeclampsia is a disease that usually happens toward the end of pregnancy and is more common among women having their first baby or women having twins or triplets. If your mother or sister had preeclampsia when she was pregnant, you have a greater chance of getting it, too. Preeclampsia can make you very sick and can make the baby sick. When preeclampsia gets really bad, it can cause the mother to have seizures. It is very important to get treatment if you have preeclampsia, so you need to call the doctor, nurse, or midwife right away if symptoms develop.

The symptoms can come on very suddenly, and can be mild or can be very strong:

- One of the first symptoms is high blood pressure. This is why your provider takes your blood pressure every time you have a prenatal visit.
- Your urine starts to have protein in it. This is one of the reasons why your provider tests your urine during prenatal care.
- You get swelling in your hands, face, or feet. Some women can't get their rings on their fingers or their shoes on their feet.
- You might have blurred vision or spots before your eyes.
- You might have a headache that won't go away.
- You might have pain under your ribs.
- You might have a sudden weight gain—maybe even 1 pound every day

If you have any of those symptoms—you don't have to have them all— call your doctor, nurse, or midwife right away and tell him or her. Don't wait until your next prenatal care visit to tell them.

Flesch-Kincaid Reading Level: 6.5

Special Instructions _____

_____

_____

_____

Phone number to call if you have questions: _____

Copyright © 2002 Lippincott Williams & Wilkins. Developed by MC Freda, EdD, RN, CHES, FAAN.

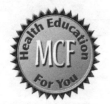

¿Qué es Preeclampsia?

A lo major nunca has escuchado esta palabra. Preeclampsia es una enfermedad que sólo sucede durante el embarazo. Las personas la conocen como "toxemia". Alrededor de 6 en cada 100 mujeres sufren de preeclampsia, así que deberías conocer de que se trata, cuales son los síntomas, y cuando deberías de llamar a tu doctor, si experimentas algunos de estos síntomas.

Preeclampsia es una enfermedad que se desarrolla hacia el final del tercer trimestre, y es muy común entre madres primerizas, o en mujeres que van a tener gemelos o trillizos. Si tu madre o hermana han tenido preeclampsia cuando estaban embarazadas, corres el riesgo de padecerla. Preeclampsia puede hacerte sentir muy enferma, y puede que el bebé nazca enfermo. Cuando la enfermedad empeora puede causar en la madre que tenga convulsiones Es muy importante obtener tratamiento, así que llama a tu doctor, enfermera o comadrona si sientes algunos de estos síntomas.

Los síntomas pueden aparecer repentinamente, y pueden ser muy ligeros o muy fuertes:

- Uno de los primeros síntomas es la presión arterial alta. Por esto es que el doctor chequea tu presión cada vez que vas a tu visita prenatal.
- La orina presenta rasgos de proteína. Esto es una de las razones por lo cual tu doctor te hace un exámen de orina durante tus visitas prenatales.
- Las manos, pies o cara se hinchan. Algunas mujeres no pueden usar sus anillos ó zapatos.
- Quizás la vista se te nuble o veas como puntitos frente tus ojos.
- Quizás tengas dolor de cabeza que no se alivia.
- Podrás sentir dolor debajo de las costillas.
- Puedes experimentar aumento de peso-hasta una libra por día.

Si tienes cualquiera de estos síntomas-no tienes que tener todos a la vez- llama a tu doctor, enfermera o comadrona de immediato e informales lo que está pasando. No esperes hasta tu próxima visita prenatal para informarles.

Special Instructions _____

_____

_____

_____

Phone number to call if you have questions: _____

Copyright © 2002 Lippincott Williams & Wilkins. Developed by MC Freda, EdD, RN, CHES, FAAN.

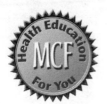

Woman's name: _____

Date: _____

Nurse's name: _____

Coping With Bed Rest

Sometimes it is suggested that pregnant women need to rest in bed due to a health problem that develops during pregnancy. This might be risk for preterm birth, or some other high-risk condition such as preeclampsia. Although many of us, in our busy lives, joke about wishing we could just stay in bed, actually bed rest can be a very difficult thing for women to endure. Being told that you cannot do all the things you usually do for yourself or for your family can be very stressful for you.

Here are some things that seem to have helped other women who are on bed rest during pregnancy:

Boredom is a major problem

- Do several different types of activities that keep your mind occupied.
- If you love to read, but never had the time, this is the time to have someone bring you all the books you have wanted to read for years!
- Even if you enjoy television, try not to spend all your time watching television. Television watching doesn't require any thought, and women who are on bed rest need to keep their minds active!
- Do you like crossword puzzles, or knitting, or sewing? This is your chance to have the time to do those things.
- Don't become isolated. Reach out to others by telephone or e-mail. If you have a computer, set it up right next to your bed, or use a laptop computer, and connect to the Internet. There are many exciting sites to see on the World Wide Web, and some are specifically for pregnant women on bed rest.

Do family chores when in bed to feel more like a member of the family

- Someone else can wash and dry the laundry, but you can fold it in bed.
- Some meal preparation such as peeling vegetables and making salad can be done in bed.
- Your other children can sit in bed with you when you help them with their homework.

Set short-term goals, and then celebrate milestones!

- Each week that passes gives your baby a better chance to be born healthy, so celebrate the end of each week with a special party every Sunday!

Connect with other women in your situation to gather support and ideas

- Use the internet to connect with www.sidelines.org and chat with other women on bed rest. Support from others can help you to cope.

    Keep remembering your goal—to have a healthy baby.
    Try to keep a positive attitude!

Flesch-Kincaid Reading Level: 7.2

Special Instructions _____

_____

Phone number to call if you have questions: _____

Copyright © 2002 Lippincott Williams & Wilkins. Developed by MC Freda, EdD, RN, CHES, FAAN.

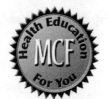

Woman's name: _____

Date: _____

Nurse's name: _____

Enfrentando el Reposo en Cama

Algunas veces se le recomienda a la mujer embarazada la necesidad de guardar reposo en cama debido a algún problema de salud que se manifestó durante el embarazo. Esto puede ser riesgoso para un parto prematuro o para otra situación de alto riesgo tal como la preeclampsia. Mientras que muchos de nosotros, durante nuestras vidas atareadas, bromeamos sobre la idea de quedarnos en cama esto puede ser en la actualidad una cosa muy difícil de tolerar para las mujeres. El que le digan a uno de que ya no puede hacer las cosas que usualmente hace por sí mismo o para su familia, puede ser de mucha tensión para la persona.

He aqui algunas de las cosas que parecen haber ayudado a otras mujeres que guardan cama durante el embarazo:

El Aburrimiento es el mayor problema.

- Realice varios tipos de actividades las cuales le mantengan la mente ocupada
- ¿Le gusta el rompecabezas, croche o cocer? Esta es su oportunidad de tener el tiempo para hacer esas cosas.
- Si le encanta leer pero nunca ha tenido el tiempo, éste es el momento de hacer que alguien le traiga todos los libros que por años usted siempre ha querido leer .
- Aunque usted disfrute ver la televisión, trate de no pasar todo su tiempo mirando televisión. El mirar televisión no le exige pensar y las mujeres que estan guardando cama necesitan mantener sus mentes activas.
- No se aislen. Comuníquese con otros por teléfono o correo electrónico. Si usted tiene una computadora colóquela junto a su cama, o use una computadora portátil o conéctese a la internet. Existen muchos sitios excitantes que ver en la red mundial y algunos de ellos son específicamente para mujeres embarazadas que guardan cama.

Realice faenas familiars mientras que esté en cama para así sentirse como un miembro de la familia.

- Otra persona puede lavar y secar la ropa, y usted puede doblarla en su cama.
- Algunos preparativos para la comida tales como pelar vegetales y preparar la ensalada se pueden hacer en la cama.
- Sus otros niños se pueden sentar en su cama con usted mientras los ayuda con sus tareas.

Fíjese objetivos a corto plazo y luego celebre los triunfos!

- Cada semana que pasa le dará a su bebé una major oportunidad de nacer saludable, así que celebre el final de cada semana con una fiesta especial todos los domingos.

Comuníquese con otras mujeres que esten en su misma situación para compartir ideas y apoyo

- Use la Internet para conectarse con www.sidelines.org y charlar con otras mujeres que esten guardando cama. El apoyo de otros le puede ayudar a afrontar la situación.

Trate de mantener una actitud positiva. Eso la mantiene saludable, y también lo puede ayudar al bebé.

Special Instructions _____

Phone number to call if you have questions: _____

Copyright © 2002 Lippincott Williams & Wilkins. Developed by MC Freda, EdD, RN, CHES, FAAN.

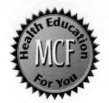

Woman's name: _____

Date: _____

Nurse's name: _____

2 Babies? 3 Babies? More?

So You're Having Multiples!!!!

It's usually a big surprise when people find out they're having more than one baby. Some people need time to get used to the idea, so don't be surprised if you need to think about this for awhile before you really accept it.

There are a lot more multiple births these days, some of them natural and some of them because of fertility drugs. **What you need to know is that a pregnancy with multiples is different from other pregnancies and has special risks.** Multiples are more likely to be born too early and too small, so you need to take special care of yourself. These are some of the things that you need to do:

- *Get good prenatal care—it's probably a good idea to see a specialist in high-risk pregnancies. You will also probably have more ultrasounds and fetal heart testing in the last few months of your pregnancy.*
- *Get extra nutrition—you need to eat well. Add about 300 more calories to your diet every day. You should discuss this with a nutritionist or your doctor, nurse, or midwife so you know what to eat.*
- *Be ready for extra weight gain—depending on how many babies you are carrying, you will probably gain about 35, 45, or more pounds.*
- *Get extra rest—you need to make time for rest during the day.*
- *Ask for help—now is the time to talk to your family about the help you will need during this pregnancy. You might need help with housework, laundry, food shopping, or babysitting for your other children.*
- *You might have extra discomforts of pregnancy like varicose veins, constipation, indigestion, heartburn, shortness of breath, or tiredness. This is common in multiple pregnancies. Tell you doctor, nurse, or midwife if these things are too uncomfortable*
- *Understand the symptoms of preterm labor—come to the hospital if you have cramps, pelvic pressure, backache, contractions, or bleeding or fluid coming from your vagina. Remember, having a multiple pregnancy puts you at high risk for preterm labor.*

Flesch-Kincaid Reading Level: 7.2

Special Instructions _____

_____

_____

_____

Phone number to call if you have questions: _____

Copyright © 2002 Lippincott Williams & Wilkins. Developed by MC Freda, EdD, RN, CHES, FAAN.

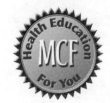

Woman's name: _____

Date: _____

Nurse's name: _____

¿¿¿¿2 Bebés???? ¿¿¿¿3 Bebés???? ¿¿Más??

¡¡¡¡Entonces Tendrás Más de Uno!!!!

Normalmente es una grande sorpresa cuando las personas se dan cuenta que tendrán más de un bebé. Algunos necesitan tiempo para acostumbrarse a la idea, bien pués no se sorprenda si tienen que pensarlo por un tiempo antes de aceptarlo.

Hay muchos más embarazos múltiples hoy en día, algunos naturales y otros a causa de medicamento para la fertilidad. **Lo que requiere saber es que el embarazo múltiple es diferente de otros embarazos y tiene riesgos especiales.** Los múltiples son más propensos a nacer más temprano y más pequeños. Asi que necesita cuidado especial. Estas son algunas cosas que debe hacer:

- *Tenga buen cuidado prenatal—es buena idea ver a un especialista en embarazos de alto riesgo. Es probable que tenga más sonogramas y pruebas del latido fetal en los últimos meses de embarazo.*
- *Obtenga nutrición extra—necesita comer bien. Agrege alrededor de 300 más calorias a su dieta diaria. Debe discutirlo con una nutricionista o su doctor, enfermera o partera para que sepa que comer*
- *Espere aumentar de peso—dependiendo de cuantos bebés esté embarazada probablemente aumente de 35, 45, o más libras.*
- *Tome descanso extra—necesita tomar tiempo durante el día para descansar*
- *Pida ayuda—ahora es el tiempo de hablarle a su familia sobre la ayuda que necesita durante el embarazo. Podría requerir ayuda con el trabajo de la casa, lavado de ropa, compra de alimentos, cuidado de sus otros niños.*
- *Podría tener molestias extras del embarazo tal como venas varicosas, estreñimiento, indigestión, reflujo esofágico, dificultad respiratoria, cansancio. Esto es común en embarazos multiples. Comuníquese con su doctor, enfermera o partera si las molestias son muy fuertes.*
- *Aprenda los síntomas de embarazo prematuro—Vaya al hospital si siente dolor, presión pélvica, dolor de espalda, contracciones, sangrado o flujo saliendo de su vagina. Recuerde que un embarazo multiple la pone en riesgo de dar a luz antes de tiempo.*

Special Instructions _____

_____

_____

Phone number to call if you have questions: _____

Copyright © 2002 Lippincott Williams & Wilkins. Developed by MC Freda, EdD, RN, CHES, FAAN.

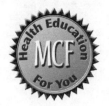

Woman's name: _____

Date: _____

Nurse's name: _____

High and Low Blood Sugar: Do You Know the Difference?

↑↑ High Blood Sugar

Why it happens

There is not enough insulin in your blood
You have an infection or fever
You have too much sugar in your diet
You are under a lot of stress

How do you know it's happening?

Increased thirst and appetite
Large amounts of sugar in the urine or blood
Ketones in the urine
Weakness, abdominal pain, generalized aches
Loss of appetite, nausea, or vomiting

What you should do?

Call your doctor, nurse, or midwife
Drink some liquid without sugar in it
Go to the hospital if your blood sugar is more than 250 or if your baby stops moving as much as normal

↓↓ Low Blood Sugar

Why it happens

There is too much insulin in your blood
You had an unusual amount of exercise
You have not eaten enough

How do you know it's happening?

Heavy sweating and feeling faint
Headache, pounding heart, trembling
Hunger, irritability
Personality changes

What you should do:

Call your doctor, nurse, or midwife
Drink some liquid with sugar in it like orange juice
Do not take any more insulin until you talk to your provider

Flesch-Kincaid Reading Level: 4.4

Special Instructions _____

_____

Phone number to call if you have questions: _____

Copyright © 2002 Lippincott Williams & Wilkins. Developed by MC Freda, EdD, RN, CHES, FAAN.

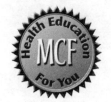

Woman's name: _____
Date: _____
Nurse's name: _____

Azúcar en la sangre (alta ó baja)
¿Sabes cuál es la diferencia?

↑↑ Azúcar en la sangre (Alta)

¿Porqué sucede?

No hay suficiente insulina en la sangre.
Tienes una infección o fiebre.
Hay mucha azúcar en tu dieta.
Tienes mucho estrés.

¿Cómo sabes que está sucediendo?

Aumento de apetito y sed.
Grandes cantidades de azúcar en la orina o sangre.
Ketones en la orina.
Debilidad , dolor abdominal, dolor generalizado.
Falta de apetito, náusea o vómito

¿Qué debes hacer?

Llamar a tu doctor, enfermera o comadrona
Tomar algun líquido con azúcar, como el jugo de naranja
Ir al hospital si el nivel de azúcar en la sangre es más de 250 ó si tu bebé para de moverse.

↓↓ Azúcar en la sangre (Baja)

¿Porqué sucede?

Hay exceso de insulina en la sangre.
Demasiado ejercicio.
No has comido lo suficiente.

¿Cómo sabes que está sucediendo?

Sudor profuso y desmayo
Dolor de cabeza, temblor, taquicardia.
Hambre, irritabilidad.
Cambios de personalidad,

¿Qué debes hacer?

Llamar a tu doctor, enfermera ó comadrona.
Tomar algun líquido con azúcar , como el jugo de naranja.
No tome más insulina hasta que hables con tu doctor.

Special Instructions _____

_____

Phone number to call if you have questions: _____

Copyright © 2002 Lippincott Williams & Wilkins. Developed by MC Freda, EdD, RN, CHES, FAAN.

Woman's name: _____

Date: _____

Nurse's name: _____

Important Information for You About Health Care Proxy, Advance Directives, and Living Wills

Because of new laws in many states, every person who goes to a hospital must be given this information. **Please Read This And Go Over It With Your Doctor, Nurse, Or Midwife.** This law says that before you are admitted to a hospital, you should choose someone you trust to make decisions about your treatment if something happens and you can't make those decisions yourself. Depending on where you live, this might be called a **"Health Care Proxy," "Advance Directive," or "Living Will."** It is very important that you think about this and talk it over with your family so you know which person you want to make health decisions for you if that becomes necessary.

Why Would You Need This?

Although it is not likely, you could become too sick to tell the doctors what you want. *If that happens, someone else has to tell them, and You Should Be The One To Choose Who That Other Person Is.* Sometimes when there is a lot of stress, like when someone is very sick, family members can't agree on what to do next. That's why it's so important that before you go into the hospital, you have made a choice about who will make health decisions for you.

How Do You Choose This Person?

There is a special paper called a "Health Care Proxy" that you will be given and asked to sign. On that paper you write the name of the person you chose and the special instructions about what you want done. If you suddenly became very sick, for instance, and you couldn't think or speak or recognize anyone, do you want machines to keep you alive? Do you want blood transfusions? Do you want liquid food by feeding tubes? These are things that are hard to think about, but very important. If you can't tell the doctors what you want, the best way to have your wishes carried out is to have the person you have chosen tell them.

Whom Should You Choose?

The best person would be a close relative like a husband, mother, father, adult child, sister or brother, or very close friend. The person must be someone you trust and must be over the age of 18.

What Happens Next?

When you go to the hospital, you will be asked to sign the form. You should keep it with you, and *Give a Copy To The Person You Chose*. Remember, even though you sign the paper, the person you chose cannot make any decisions for you unless you cannot make decisions yourself. As long as you are okay, you will make your own decisions about your health care.

Flesch-Kincaid Reading Level: 6.4

Special Instructions _____

_____

Phone number to call if you have questions: _____

Copyright © 2002 Lippincott Williams & Wilkins. Developed by MC Freda, EdD, RN, CHES, FAAN.

Información Importante Para Usted "Health Care Proxy", "Advance Directive", "Living Will"

Por una nueva ley en muchos estados, a cada persona que vaya a un hospital debe dársele esta informacíon. **Favor lea esto y revíselo con su doctor, enfermera o partera**. Esta ley dice que antes de que sea admitida al Hospital, usted debe escoger a alguien de su confianza para tomar decisiones acerca de su tratamiento si algo pasa y usted no pueda hacer esa decisión por sí misma. Dependiendo de donde viva esta ley puede llamarse **"Health Care Proxy," "Advance Directive," o "Living Will."** Es muy importante, piense sobre esto y hable con su familia para escoger que persona quiere que tome decisiones de salud por usted si fuera necesario.

¿Porqué necesita esto?

Aunque sea improbable, usted podría estar tan enferma que no pueda decirle al doctor lo que quiera. **Si esto sucede, otra persona tiene que decirle, y Usted Debe Escoger Quien Seria Esa Otra Persona.** En ocasiones cuando hay mucho estrés, como cuando alguien está muy enfermo, los miembros de la familia no pueden acordar que hacer. Por eso es tan importante que antes que vaya al hospital, decida quien vaya a tomar decision de salud por usted.

¿Como escoger esa persona?

Hay un papel especial llamado "Health Care Proxy"el cual se le pedirá que firme. En ese papel escriba el nombre de la persona escogida, e instrucciones especiales acerca de que quiere que se haga. Si llega a estar muy enferma, y en caso de que no pueda hablar, pensar o reconocer a alguien, ¿quiere que máquinas la mantengan viva? ¿Quiere transfusiones de sangre? ¿Quiere alimentación liquída por tubos? Hay cosas que son difícil de imaginar, pero son muy importantes.

Si no quiere decirle al doctor lo que quiere, lo mejor es dejar que la persona que usted eligió le comunique sus deseos al doctor.

¿A Quien Debe Escoger?

La mejor persona es un familiar cercano como su esposo, mamá, papá, hijo adulto, hermana ó hermano o un amigo cercano. La persona debe ser alguien en quien confíe y de edad mayor de 18.

¿Qué Pasa Luego?

Cuando vaya al hospital, le pedirán que firme el formulario. Quédese con el **y Dele Una Copia A La Persona Que Ha Escogido**. Recuerde, aunque ha firmado el papel la persona escogida no puede tomar decisión por usted, a menos que no pueda hacerlas por sí misma. Mientras se encuentre bien, usted hará sus propias decisiones sobre su salud.

Special Instructions _____

_____

_____

Phone number to call if you have questions: _____

Copyright © 2002 Lippincott Williams & Wilkins. Developed by MC Freda, EdD, RN, CHES, FAAN.

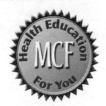

Woman's name: _____

Date: _____

Nurse's name: _____

Heparin Use in Pregnancy

Although we tell pregnant women not to take any drugs during pregnancy, sometimes it is necessary to take certain medicines during pregnancy that are prescribed by your provider.

What Is Heparin?

Heparin is a medicine that can help to thin the blood and prevent blood clots from forming where they shouldn't. The most common place for a blood clot to form is in your leg. A blood clot in your leg can be dangerous, because it can break loose and travel to other parts of your body—this can cause serious damage. A clot in the lung can cause problems breathing, and can be dangerous for you and for the baby. Heparin can help to prevent a clot, and if your provider has told you that you already have a clot, heparin can keep the clot from getting bigger. Heparin is given in a shot, once or twice a day.

Who Needs Heparin?

Heparin is only given when a health care provider prescribes it. It could be prescribed for a woman who has had a blood clot in her leg in the past, or for a woman who has a blood clot in her leg right now, or for a woman who has a blood clot in her lung.

How Do I Take the Heparin?

Your nurse will teach you how to give yourself shots of Heparin. *It is very important that you do not take any aspirin if you are using Heparin.*

Are There Any Problems With Taking Heparin?

If you take heparin and any of the following things happen to you, call your health care provider right away:

Bleeding from your gums
Black and blue marks on your body
Nosebleeds
Blood in your urine
Black tarry stools

   Be Sure To Call Your Doctor, Nurse, Or Midwife If You Have Any Questions Or Problems With Your Heparin.

Flesch-Kincaid Reading Level: 5.9

Special Instructions _____

Phone number to call if you have questions: _____

Copyright © 2002 Lippincott Williams & Wilkins. Developed by MC Freda, EdD, RN, CHES, FAAN.

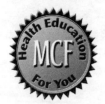

Woman's name: _____
Date: _____
Nurse's name: _____

Heparina Usada En El Embarazo

Aunque le decimos a las mujeres embarazadas que no usen medicamentos durante el embarazo a veces es necesario tomar ciertos medicamentos durante el embarazo si son recetados por su proveedor de salud.

¿Qué Es Heparina?

La heparina es un medicamento que ayuda a hacer a la sangre menos espesa y previene la producción de coágulos donde no deberían existir. El lugar más común para la formación de coágulos de sangre es en las piernas. Un coágulo de sangre en una pierna es peligroso porque puede romperse y moverse a otras partes de su cuerpo - esto puede causar serio daño. Un coágulo de sangre en sus pulmones puede causarle problemas para la respiración, y podría ser peligroso para usted y para su bebé. La heparina puede ayudarle a prevenir un coágulo y si su proveedor le ha indicado que ya tiene uno, la heparina puede prevenir su crecimiento. La heparina es dada a través de una inyección una o dos veces al día.

¿Quién Necesita Heparina?

Heparina solo es dada cuando un proveedor de salud la receta. Puede ser recetada para una mujer con historia de coágulos en el pasado, o para una mujer que tenga coágulos en las piernas, o para una que lo tenga en los pulmones.

¿Cómo Uso La Heparina?

Su enfermera le mostrará como puede darse a sí misma las inyecciones de Heparina.
   Es muy importante que no tome aspirina si está usando Heparina.

¿Hay Algun Problema Al Tomar Heparina?

Si toma Heparina y algunas de estas cosas le suceden, llame a su proveedor de salud de inmediato:

Sangrado de las encías
Manchas negras o azules en su cuerpo
Sangrado nasal
Sangre en la orina
Heces obscuras o negras

   Asegúrese de llamar a su doctor, enfermera, o partera si tiene cualquier pregunta o problemas con la heparina

Special Instructions _____

Phone number to call if you have questions: _____

Copyright © 2002 Lippincott Williams & Wilkins. Developed by MC Freda, EdD, RN, CHES, FAAN.

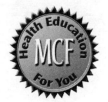

Woman's name: _____

Date: _____

Nurse's name: _____

Yeast Infections and How to Cure Them

Why Do Women Get Yeast Infections??

Yeast infections are very common in women and are caused by something called *Candida* growing too fast in your vagina. Yeast infections can happen after a woman has taken antibiotics for another type of infection, during pregnancy, to women who are diabetics, or to women who wear tight jeans or other tight clothing that holds in moisture.

How Do I Know If I Have a Yeast Infection??

If you have a vaginal discharge and you are very itchy and red around your vagina, you probably have a yeast infection. You should see a health care provider if you think you have a yeast infection so you can be given the right medicine.

How Do I Get Rid of a Yeast Infection??

There are a few different treatments. You will probably be given a medicine that you need to put into your vagina. Sometimes the treatment takes 7 days, and sometimes less, but your doctor, nurse, or midwife should explain exactly how to use the medicine and for how long. **You must use the medicine just as they tell you to, because the yeast infection will come right back unless the medicine is used correctly.** If your partner has any itching or redness around his penis, he should see a health care provider and be treated, too.

If you are thinking of just going to a drug store and buying medicine, you should really talk to your provider first to make sure you have a yeast infection. It isn't a good idea to use medicine if you're not sure what the infection is.

How Can I Prevent Another Yeast Infection??

Sometimes these infections cannot be prevented, but there are a few things that you can do:

- *Always wipe from front to back after going to the bathroom.*
- *Don't wear tight jeans, underwear, or panty hose for too many hours at a time. Tight clothes don't let any air get to your vaginal area.*
- *Don't use any douches unless your provider has told you to.*

Be Sure To Ask Your Doctor, Nurse, Or Midwife About This.

Flesch-Kincaid Reading Level: 7.5

Special Instructions _____

Phone number to call if you have questions: _____

Copyright © 2002 Lippincott Williams & Wilkins. Developed by MC Freda, EdD, RN, CHES, FAAN.

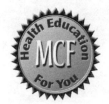

Woman's name: _____
Date: _____
Nurse's name: _____

Infecciones Por Hongos Y Como Curarlas

¿¿Porqué Las Mujeres Adquieren Infecciones Por Hongos??

Las infecciones por hongos son muy comunes en mujeres, y son causadas por algo llamado **Candida** creciendo muy rápido en su vagina. Infecciones por hongos suceden después que la mujer ha tomado antibióticos por otro tipo de infección, durante el embarazo, en mujeres que son diabéticas o en mujeres que usan jeans u otra ropa muy apretadas y húmedas.

¿¿Cómo Sé Si Tengo Una Infección Por Hongo??

Si tiene flujo vaginal, si tiene picazón y enrojecimiento alrededor de la vagina, es probable que tenga una infección por hongo. Debe ver un proveedor de salud si cree tener una infección por hongo para que reciba el medicamento adecuado.

¿¿Cómo Me Curo De Una Infección Por Hongo??

Hay diferentes tratamientos. Es probable que le den medicamentos que tenga que aplicarse en su vagina. A veces el tratamiento dura 7 días o menos, pero su doctor enfermera o partera debe explicarle como usar el medicamento y por cuanto tiempo. **Usted debe usar el medicamento tal y como se le indique, de lo contrario la infección regresará si no es usado correctamente.** Si su pareja tiene picazón o enrojecimiento en su pene él debe ir al proveedor de salud y ser tratado.

Si está pensando solo ir a la farmacia y comprar medicina, debería ir primero a su proveedor de salud y asegurarse si tiene una infección por hongo. No es buena idea usar medicamentos sin estar segura que tipo de infección tenga.

¿¿Cómo Puedo Prevenir Otra Infección Por Hongo??

A veces estas infecciones no pueden prevenirse , pero hay algunas cosas que puede hacer

- *Siempre límpiese de adelante hacia atrás después de ir al baño*
- *No use jeans o ropa interior apretada por muchas horas seguidas esto no permite al aire llegar a su área vaginal*
- *No use duchas vaginales si no es indicado por su proveedor de salud*

Asegurese De Preguntarle A Su Doctor, Enfermera O Partera Al Respecto.

Special Instructions _____

_____

Phone number to call if you have questions:_____

Copyright © 2002 Lippincott Williams & Wilkins. Developed by MC Freda, EdD, RN, CHES, FAAN.

Woman's name: _____
Date: _____
Nurse's name: _____

Diabetes in Pregnancy (Gestational Diabetes)

What Is Diabetes in Pregnancy?

When you have diabetes, your body doesn't use sugar the way it is supposed to. Normally when you eat, your body makes insulin to help use the sugar for energy. For some pregnant women, the hormones of pregnancy keep your body from using insulin, and then you develop diabetes in pregnancy (also called gestational diabetes). When this happens, your blood sugar goes too high. This can affect the growth of your baby.

What Are the Dangers of Diabetes in Pregnancy?

A large baby that is hard to deliver
A greater chance of cesarean birth
Possible health problems with your newborn right after birth

Why Did You Get Diabetes in Pregnancy?

You didn't cause the diabetes. It happens to many women, and no one really understands why some women get it and other women don't. When you are told that you have diabetes in pregnancy you might feel sad or angry, and you might ask "Why me?" Most women feel that way. Just remember that diabetes in pregnancy is a condition that can be treated. By following directions and taking good care of yourself during your pregnancy you will have a very good chance of having a healthy baby.

How Can You Best Take Care of Yourself With Diabetes in Pregnancy?

It is most important that you learn how to check your blood sugar and eat the right foods when you have diabetes in pregnancy. This will help you and your baby. Your doctor, nurse, or midwife will teach you about how to take care of yourself during this pregnancy. Ask him or her as many questions as you need to.

These Are Some of the Things That Can Help Keep You and Your Baby Healthy

Don't miss any of your prenatal or fetal testing appointments
Follow the diet you are given (don't skip meals or snacks)
Learn everything you can about diabetes in pregnancy
Test your blood sugar as directed
Take insulin as your doctor, nurse, or midwife teaches you

Flesch-Kincaid Reading Level: 5.7

Special Instructions _____

_____

Phone number to call if you have questions: _____

Copyright © 2002 Lippincott Williams & Wilkins. Developed by MC Freda, EdD, RN, CHES, FAAN.

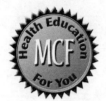

Woman's name: _____
Date: _____
Nurse's name: _____

Diabetes Gestacional

¿Qué Es la Diabetes Del Embarazo?

Cuando tiene Diabetes, su cuerpo no usa el azúcar en la forma en que está supuesto. Normalmente cuando come, su cuerpo produce Insulina para ayudar a usar el azúcar como energía. Para algunas mujeres embarazadas, las hormonas del embarazo impiden el uso correcto de la Insulina, entonces desarrollan Diabetes Del Embarazo (también llamado Diabetes Gestacional). Esto aumenta el azúcar sanguínea y puede afectar el crecimiento del bebé

¿Cuáles Son Los Peligros De La Diabetes Del Embarazo?

Un bebé muy grande y difícil de parir
Un mayor chance de Cesárea
Posible problemas del bebé al nacer

¿Porqué Adquirió Diabetes Del Embarazo?

Usted no causó la Diabetes. Sucede a muchas mujeres y ninguna realmente entiende porque algunas mujeres la adquieren y otras no. Cuando dicen que tiene Diabetes Del Embarazo podría sentirse triste, o enfadada y podría preguntarse "¿porqué a mi?" la mayoría de las mujeres se sienten así. Sólo recuerde que la Diabetes Del Embarazo es una condición que puede ser tratada. Tomando buen cuidado de sí misma y siguiendo instrucciones tiene buen chance de tener un bebé saludable.

¿Cómo Puede Cuidarse Si Tiene Diabetes Del Embarazo?

Lo más importante es que aprenda a chequear la glucosa sanguínea y coma los alimentos apropiados si tiene Diabetes Del Embarazo. Esto ayudará a su bebé. Su doctor, enfermera o partera le instruirá de como cuidarse durante el embarazo. Pregúntele todas las preguntas que quiera.

Estas Son Algunas Cosas Que Pueden Mantenerla Saludable A Usted Y Su Bebé:

No falte a ninguna cita prenatal o cita de prueba fetal
Siga la dieta que se le dé (no omita comidas o picaderas)
Aprenda todo lo que pueda sobre Diabetes Del Embarazo
Chequee su azúcar en la sangre como se le indique
Tome la Insulina como su doctor, enfermera o partera le indique

Special Instructions _____

_____

Phone number to call if you have questions: _____

Copyright © 2002 Lippincott Williams & Wilkins. Developed by MC Freda, EdD, RN, CHES, FAAN.

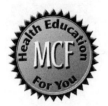

Woman's name: _____

Date: _____

Nurse's name: _____

Your Body Needs Iron

What Is Iron, and Why Do I Need to Take It??

Iron is a mineral that everyone needs to stay healthy. Women who are pregnant or who were recently pregnant need iron even more than other people. This is because your body uses iron to make more blood when you are pregnant.

What Is Iron Deficiency??

You can develop *Iron deficiency (also called "Anemia")* when you don't get enough iron. This can make you feel tired, you can get colds or the flu more easily, you can lose weight, or you may not feel like eating.

What Do I Do If I Have Iron Deficiency??

The best thing to do if you have iron deficiency is to eat lots of foods that have iron in them. These are the foods that you should be eating:

Lean Red Meat	*Peanut Butter*	*Vegetables*
Sardines	*Oatmeal*	*Dried Fruit*
Whole Wheat Bread	*Green Beans*	*Brown Rice*

What Else Should I Do?

If you are given iron pills to take, be sure to take them every day.
Try not to drink coffee or tea. Coffee and tea make it harder for your body to use the iron you eat in your food.

Try to eat lots of foods with vitamin C in them, like oranges, grapefruits, broccoli, melons, mustard greens, collards, and kale. The vitamin C helps your body to use the iron better.

Ask Your Doctor, Nurse, Or Midwife If You Have Questions About This.

Flesch-Kincaid Reading Level: 6.9

Special Instructions _____

_____

_____

_____

Phone number to call if you have questions: _____

Copyright © 2002 Lippincott Williams & Wilkins. Developed by MC Freda, EdD, RN, CHES, FAAN.

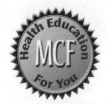

Woman's name: _____
Date: _____
Nurse's name: _____

Su Cuerpo Necesita Hierro

¿¿Qué Es Hierro, Y Porque Necesito Tomarlo??

Hierro es un mineral que todos necesitamos para mantenernos en buena salud. Las mujeres embarazadas o que lo han estado recientemente necesitan más hierro que otras personas, porque su cuerpo usa más hierro para hacer sangre durante el embarazo.

¿¿Qué Es La Deficiencia Del Hierro??

Usted puede desarrollar **Deficiencia de Hierro (también llamada "Anemia")** cuando usted no consume suficiente hierro. Esto puede hacerla sentir cansada o podría darle la gripe, pérdida de peso o pérdida de apetito.

¿¿Qué Hacer Si Tiene Deficiencia De Hierro??

Lo mejor que pueda hacer si tiene deficiencia de hierro es comer más alimentos que contengan hierro. Estos son los alimentos que deberías comer:

Carne Roja	*Mantequilla De Maní*	*Vegetales*
Sardinas	*Avena*	*Frutas Frescas*
Pan Integral	*Habichuelas Verdes*	*Arroz Integral*

¿¿Qué más debo hacer??

Si le dan pastillas de hierro para tomar, no olvide tomarlas todos los días.
Trate de no tomar café o té. Esto dificulta que el bebé use el hierro que usted consuma en las comidas.

Trata de comer muchos alimentos con vitamina C, tales como: naranjas, toronjas, brocoli, melones, mostaza, y col rizada. La vitamina C ayuda a su cuerpo a usar mejor el hierro consumido.

Si Tiene Otra Pregunta Sobre Esto Pregúntele A Su Doctor, Enfermera O Partera

Special Instructions _____

_____

_____

_____

Phone number to call if you have questions: _____

Copyright © 2002 Lippincott Williams & Wilkins. Developed by MC Freda, EdD, RN, CHES, FAAN.

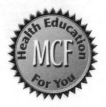

Woman's name: _____

Date: _____

Nurse's name: _____

Colposcopy

You are scheduled to have a special test called a "colposcopy." This should answer some questions you might have.

What Is a Colposcopy???

A "colposcopy" (pronounced "coll-poss-co-pee") is a test done by a doctor, midwife, or nurse. It is done as a part of a pelvic exam, using a kind of microscope called a "colposcope." When doing the pelvic exam, the provider can look through the colposcope to see a larger view of your vagina and cervix (the neck of your womb). This test does not hurt. It is like a regular pelvic exam, but it takes a little longer.

Why Do I Need a Colposcopy?

Colposcopy is usually ordered because your last Pap test was not normal. This means that some cells from your cervix looked abnormal and need to be checked out further. This does not necessarily mean that there is something wrong with you; it just means that another test should be done to understand what is happening.

Does This Mean That I Have Cancer?

No it does not mean that you have cancer, but it is very important that this test is done so that if <u>anything</u> is wrong it can be treated right away. If any abnormal cells are seen during the test, then a biopsy (removing a small piece of tissue) will be done. You might feel some cramps during the biopsy.

What Happens After the Colposcopy Test Is Over?

On your next visit to the doctor, nurse, or midwife he or she will discuss all the results with you. He or she will help to plan what needs to be done next.

<u>It is very important that you come to the next visit and that you have a regular Pap test every 6 months to 1 year from now on.</u>

Flesch-Kincaid Reading Level: 6.2

Special Instructions _____

_____

_____

_____

_____

Phone number to call if you have questions: _____

Copyright © 2002 Lippincott Williams & Wilkins. Developed by MC Freda, EdD, RN, CHES, FAAN.

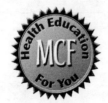

Woman's name: _____
Date: _____
Nurse's name: _____

Colposcopía

*Usted tiene una cita para una prueba especial llamada "colposcopía".
Esto prodría responder algunas preguntas que usted tenga.*

¿¿¿Qué Es Una Colposcopía???

Una "colposcopía" es un prueba hecha por el doctor, enfermera o partera. Es una parte del exámen pélvico, usando una forma de microscopio llamado "colposcopio". Durante el exámen el examinador puede ver a través del colposcopio y tener una vista de su vagina y cervix (el cuello del útero). Esta prueba no duele. Es como un examen pélvico regular, pero toma un poco más de tiempo.

¿Porqué Necesito Una Colposcopía?

La colposcopía es usualmente indicada si su última prueba de Pap no es normal, esto significa que las células de su cervix lucen anormal y requieren más chequeo. Esto no significa necesariamente que tenga algo malo, solo indica que otra prueba es requerida para investigar que está pasando.

¿Esto Significa Que Tengo Cancer?

No, no significa que usted tenga cancer, pero es muy importante que esta prueba sea hecha para que <u>cualquier cosa</u> que esté mal pueda ser tratada de inmediato. Si cualquier célula anormal es vista durante la prueba, entonces una biopsia (tomar un poquito de tejido) es hecha. Usted podría sentir alguna molestia durante la biopsia

¿Qué Pasa Después Del Exámen De La Colposcopía?

En su próxima visita con el doctor, enfermera ó partera ellos discutirán el resultado con usted. Le ayudarán a planear lo siguiente que se necesitará hacer.

<u>**Es muy importante que venga a la próxima visita, y que tenga una prueba de Pap regular cada seis a doce meses desde ahora en adelante.**</u>

Special Instructions _____

_____

_____

_____

_____

_____

Phone number to call if you have questions: _____

Copyright © 2002 Lippincott Williams & Wilkins. Developed by MC Freda, EdD, RN, CHES, FAAN.

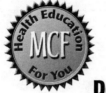

Woman's name: _____

Date: _____

Nurse's name: _____

Do You Know About Lead Poisoning and What It Can Do to Newborn Babies???

Lead poisoning can be a big problem for pregnant women and for their babies. If a pregnant woman is exposed to too much lead (like in paint, or in water, or in some herbs), that lead can be passed to her baby, and can cause the baby's brain to become damaged. Children who are exposed to lead could have problems with mental retardation. It is very important that all pregnant women and mothers know if they might be at risk for lead poisoning.

Read This List And Answer The Questions. If You Answer "Yes" To Any Of The Questions, Tell Your Doctor, Nurse, or Midwife Who May Suggest A Special Blood Test For You:

1. Do you or does anyone in your house work in a place where they are exposed to lead (painting, chemicals, auto repair, work with guns, pottery)? __Yes __No
2. Do you ever eat things that are not food (such as clay, soil, plaster, or paint chips) ? __Yes __No
3. Do you live in an old house or apartment with peeling paint or in a place with work going on that causes a lot of dust? __Yes __No
4. Have you ever been told that the water in your house or apartment has a high lead level? __Yes __No
5. Do you use any traditional folk treatments or herbs that are not sold in a regular store (kohl, surma, rauda, liga, bali goli, ghazard, greta, pay-loo-ah)? __Yes __No
6. Do you or does anyone in your house have a hobby that could use lead (making stained glass, making pottery, making jewelry, glassblowing, target shooting, making lead figurines, playing games with lead figurines)? __Yes __No
7. Do you use homemade pottery or leaded crystal? __Yes __No

Lead Poisoning Is Serious. Tell Us If There Is Any Chance You Have Been Exposed To Lead.

Flesch-Kincaid Reading Level: 4.3

Special Instructions _____

_____

_____

_____

Phone number to call if you have questions: _____

Copyright © 2002 Lippincott Williams & Wilkins. Developed by MC Freda, EdD, RN, CHES, FAAN.

Health Education For You MCF

¿¿¿Sabes Acerca Del Envenenaminto Con Plomo Y Como Puede Afectar Al Bebé???

El envenenamiento con plomo puede ser un gran problema para la mujer embarazada así como para sus bebés. Si una mujer embarazada está expuesta a mucho plomo (como en pintura o en agua) ese plomo puede pasar al bebé y causar daño al cerebro del bebé. Los niños que han sido expuestos al plomo pueden tener problemas de retraso mental. Es muy importante que todas las mujeres embarazadas y madres sepan si están en riesgo de envenenamiento con plomo.

Lea Esta Lista Y Conteste Las Preguntas. Si Su Respuesta Es "Sí" A Cualquier Pregunta, Dígale A Su Doctor, Enfermera o Partera Quien Podría Sugerir Que Se Haga Una Prueba Especial De Sangre

1. Trabaja usted o alguien en su casa en un lugar donde esté expuesta a plomo (pintura, químicos, reparación de autos, trabajo con pistolas)? __ Sí__No
2. En algun momento ha comido algo que no sea comida (como arcilla, tierra, emplasto o pintura seca)? __Si__No
3. Vive usted en casa o apartamento viejo con pintura despegada, o en un lugar donde hay trabajo que cause mucho polvo? __Sí__No
4. Le han dicho alguna vez que el agua de su casa ó apartamento tiene alto nivel de plomo? __Sí__No
5. Usa usted remedios tradicionales o hierbas que no sean vendidas en tiendas regulares(kohl, surma, rauda, liga, boli goli, ghazard, greta, pay-loo-ah)? __Sí__No
6. Tiene usted o alguien en su casa un pasatiempo el cual pueda contener plomo (pintar cristales, hacer joyas, soplar botellas, tiro al blanco, hacer figuras de plomo, jugar con figura de plomo)? __Sí__No
7. Usted usa utencilios hechos en casa o cristal con plomo? __Sí__No

El Envenenamiento Con Plomo Es Serio. Infórmanos Si Hay Alguna Posibilidad Que Haya Sido Expuesta Al Plomo.

Special Instructions _____

_____

_____

_____

_____

Phone number to call if you have questions: _____

Copyright © 2002 Lippincott Williams & Wilkins. Developed by MC Freda, EdD, RN, CHES, FAAN.

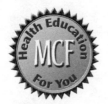

Woman's name: _____

Date: _____

Nurse's name: _____

Genetic Testing in Pregnancy

There are several tests that your doctor, nurse, or midwife may recommend during pregnancy that examine genes and chromosomes. Genetic tests look for things that are passed from generation to generation.

Amniocentesis

Amniocentesis (pronounced "am-nee-o-sen-teesis") is a test in which a small amount of amniotic fluid is removed from the uterus to examine the baby's chromosomes. It is done around 14 to 16 weeks of pregnancy. A very thin needle is put in your abdomen and a small amount of fluid from around the baby is taken out. Down syndrome and other genetic problems can be diagnosed with amniocentesis. When you have this test, the risk of a miscarriage is about 1%.

Amniocentesis may be recommended by your doctor, nurse, or midwife because you are over 35 years old (some genetic diseases are more common in older women) or because of something in your family history. You will probably be asked to see a genetic counselor before the test, who should answer all your questions. This test is voluntary. You have to agree to have the test. Speak to your doctor, nurse, or midwife about this.

Chorionic Villus Sampling (CVS)

This advantage of this test (pronounced "core-ee-on-ik vill-us") is that it can be done earlier than an amniocentesis (between the 10th and 12th weeks of pregnancy). That way, if there is something wrong, you would know earlier and could make decisions about the pregnancy earlier. In this test, a sample of the placenta (called chorionic villi), is taken either through the abdomen with a needle or through the vagina. These villi can be analyzed for genetic diseases. The miscarriage rate is about 1%. This test is also voluntary, and you do not have to have it unless you agree to it. Speak to your doctor, nurse, or midwife about this.

If your doctor, nurse, or midwife recommends genetic tests, be sure to ask questions and see a genetic counselor.

Flesch-Kincaid Reading Level: 9.0

Special Instructions _____

_____

_____

Phone number to call if you have questions: _____

Copyright © 2002 Lippincott Williams & Wilkins. Developed by MC Freda, EdD, RN, CHES, FAAN.

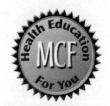

Woman's name: _____

Date: _____

Nurse's name: _____

Pruebas Genéticas durante el Embarazo

Hay varios exámenes que tu doctor, enfermera o comadrona recomendarán que te hagas durante el embarazo, los cuales examinan los genes y los cromasomas. Las pruebas genéticas localizan "cosas" que son transmitidas de generación a generación.

Amniocentesis

Amniocentesis es un exámen en el cual una pequeña cantidad del líquido amniótico es extraído del útero, para analizar los cromosomas del bebé. Este exámen es hecho cerca de las 14 o 16 semanas de gestación. Una aguja muy fina es insertada en el abdomen y una cantidad muy pequeña del líquido alrededor del bebé es extraída. El síndrome de Down y otros problemas genéticos pueden ser diagnosticados a través de la amniocentesis. El riesgo de aborto durante este exámen es cerca de 1%.

La prueba de amniocentesis es recomendada por tu doctor, enfermera o comadrona si eres mayor de 35 años (algunas enfermedades genéticas son más comunes en las mujeres mayores), o si existe algo en la historia familiar. Quizás te pedirán que veas a un consejero de genética antes del exámen. El responderá a todas tus preguntas. Este exámen es voluntario. Tienes que estar de acuerdo para el procedimiento. Consulta con tu doctor, enfermera o comadrona sobre ésto.

Prueba del Vello Coriónico (CVS)

La ventaja de esta prueba, es que puede ser hecho más temprano que la amniocentesis (entre la 10ma y 12va semana de embarazo). De esta forma si existiera algo malo, usted podría saber con tiempo suficiente y podría tomar decisiones acerca de su embarazo. En este exámen, una muestra de la placenta es extraída a través del abdomen ó de la vagina , utilizando una aguja. Esta vellosidad es analizada para detectar enfermedades genéticas. El riesgo de aborto al hacerse esta prueba es de 1%. Este exámen es voluntario, y no tienes que hacértelo, a menos que estés de acuerdo. Habla con tu doctor, enfermera o comadrona sobre esto.

Si tu doctor, enfermera, o comadrona recomiendan que te hagas éstas pruebas genéticas, asegúrate de hacer preguntas y visita a un consejero de genética.

Special Instructions _____

_____

_____

Phone number to call if you have questions: _____

Copyright © 2002 Lippincott Williams & Wilkins. Developed by MC Freda, EdD, RN, CHES, FAAN.

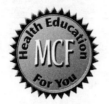

Woman's name: _____

Date: _____

Nurse's name: _____

Fibroids—What Are They?

Fibroids are extra growths in the uterus (womb). Some people call them "fibroid tumors." **They are not cancer.** They can grow inside the uterus or on the outside of the uterus. Fibroids are very common. No one knows what causes them, but they seem to run in families.

What Are The Symptoms??? Do I Have Fibroids???

Fibroids are usually found when you have a pelvic exam by a health care provider. Sometimes they can be seen during an "ultrasound" (also called "sonogram"). If the fibroids are small, there may be no symptoms. If the fibroids grow larger, these things might happen:

- **Heavy, frequent, painful periods**
- **Pain or "fullness" in the abdomen**
- **Back pain**
- **Frequent urination from pressure on the bladder**
- **Difficulty getting pregnant**

What Is the Treatment for Fibroids??

There are a few different things that might be done about fibroids:

1. **No Treatment**—If the fibroids are small, no treatment is necessary except a pelvic exam every 6 months to check on the fibroids. Sometimes fibroids get smaller when a woman reaches menopause. If this happens, no treatment is needed.
2. **Surgery to Remove the Fibroids**—This is called a "myomectomy" (pronounced MY-O-MECK-TOE-ME). This may be done when fibroids are causing symptoms and the woman wants to still be able to become pregnant.
3. **Surgery to Remove the Uterus**—This is called a "hysterectomy" (pronounced HIST-ER-ECK-TOE-ME), and if it is done you will not have menstrual periods anymore, and you can no longer have children. This is done when the symptoms of the fibroids are severe.
4. **Hormone Treatment**—Sometimes hormones can be given to shrink the size of the fibroids. This may be before a woman with large fibroids has surgery.

Be sure to ask your doctor, nurse, or midwife about the best treatment for you.

Flesch-Kincaid Reading Level: 5.1

Special Instructions _____

_____

Phone number to call if you have questions: _____

Copyright © 2002 Lippincott Williams & Wilkins. Developed by MC Freda, EdD, RN, CHES, FAAN.

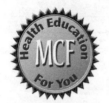

Woman's name: _____

Date: _____

Nurse's name: _____

Los Fibromas—¿Qué son?

Los Fibromas son crecimientos extras del útero(matriz). Algunas personas los llaman "tumores fibromas." **No son cancer**. Pueden crecer dentro del útero o fuera del útero. Los fibromas son muy comunes. Nadie sabe que los producen, pero parecen poder pasarse de familia a familia.

¿¿¿CUALES SON LOS SINTOMAS??? ¿¿¿TENGO FIBROMAS???

Los fibromas nomalmente se encuentran cuando un proveedor de salud le hace un examén pélvico. Algunas veces se pueden ver durante un "sonograma" . Si los fibromas son pequeños, pueda que no haya síntomas. Si los fibromas crecen más grande, estas cosas pueden ocurrir:

- **Fuertes, frecuentes y dolorosas menstruaciones**
- **Dolor o sensación de estar llena en el abdomen**
- **Dolor de espalda**
- **Frecuente orina a causa de presión en la vejiga**
- **Dificultad para embarazarse**

¿¿Cuál Es El Tratamiento Para Los Fibromas??

Hay algunas cosas diferentes que se pueden hacer sobre los fibromas:

1. **Ningún tratramiento**—Si los fibromas son pequeños, ningún tratamiento es necesario excepto por el examen pélvico cada 6 meses para evaluar los fibromas. Algunas veces los fibromas se hacen más pequeños cuando la mujer llega a la menopausa. Si esto ocurre, ningún tratamiento es necesario.
2. **Cirugía Para Remover Los Fibromas**—Esto es llamado "miomectomía." Esto es hecho cuando los fibromas están causando síntomas y la mujer todavía quiere embarazarse.
3. **Cirugía Para Remover El Utero**—Esto es llamado "histerectomía" y si esto es hecho, usted ya no tendrá su menstruación, y no podrá tener hijos. Esto es hecho cuando los síntomas de los fibromas son muy fuertes.
4. **Tratameinto de Hormonas**—Algunas veces hormonas son dadas para reducir el tamaño de los fibromas. Esto se puede hacer antes que la mujer con fibromas grandes tenga la cirugía.

Asegúrese de preguntar a su doctor, enfermera o partera sobre el mejor tratamiento para usted.

Special Instructions _____

_____

Phone number to call if you have questions: _____

Copyright © 2002 Lippincott Williams & Wilkins. Developed by MC Freda, EdD, RN, CHES, FAAN.

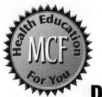

Woman's name: _____
Date: _____
Nurse's name: _____

Do You Need to Have a Vaccination for Rubella?

Before you become pregnant it's a good idea to have a blood test to find out if you need the rubella vaccine. The vaccine could keep you from getting rubella during pregnancy.

"Rubella" is also called "German measles." It is a mild disease in children, but if a pregnant woman gets it, her unborn baby can become very sick. If an unborn baby gets rubella, he or she could become deaf, be mentally retarded, have heart problems, or even die.

You can't get the vaccine while you're pregnant.
You have to get it before you get pregnant.

If you are thinking about getting pregnant, be sure you get a blood test for rubella and a vaccination if you need it at least 3 months before you get pregnant.

Talk to your doctor, your nurse, or your midwife about this.

Flesch-Kincaid Reading Level:6.9

Special Instructions _____

_____

_____

_____

_____

_____

_____

_____

Phone number to call if you have questions: _____

Copyright © 2002 Lippincott Williams & Wilkins. Developed by MC Freda, EdD, RN, CHES, FAAN.

Woman's name: _____

Date: _____

Nurse's name: _____

¿Necesita usted una vacuna contra el sarampión?

Antes de salir embarazada es una buena idea de hacerse un exámen de sangre para averiguar si necesita la vacuna contra el sarampión. La vacuna puede evitar de que le dé el sarampión durante el embarazo.

Al sarampión se le conoce también como la Rubeóla. Es una leve enfermedad entre los niños. Pero si una mujer embarazada lo contrae, su bebé en gestión se puede enfermar severamente. Sí un bebé en gestión contrae el sarampión, podría nacer sordo, ser un retardado mental, tener problemas del corazón o inclusive puede morir.

**Usted no se puede vacunar mientras está embarazada.
Tiene que vacunarse antes de salir embarazada.**

Sí usted está pensando en salir embarazada asegúrese de hacerse un exámen de sangre contra el sarampión y ponerse una vacuna si lo necesita por lo menos tres meses antes de salir embarazada.

Converse sobre ésto con su doctor, su enfermera o su comadrona.

Special Instructions _____

_____

_____

_____

_____

_____

_____

Phone number to call if you have questions: _____

Copyright © 2002 Lippincott Williams & Wilkins. Developed by MC Freda, EdD, RN, CHES, FAAN.

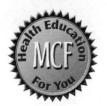

Woman's name: _____

Date: _____

Nurse's name: _____

HIV Infection and AIDS

All providers of prenatal care should talk about HIV testing with pregnant women. You might have questions about this as well. Read this handout, and then talk to your doctor, nurse, or midwife.

Could my baby be born with AIDS?

If you are infected with the HIV virus, there is about a 50% chance that your baby will also be infected. There have been recent studies that show that if you have the HIV virus and you are given medicine during your pregnancy, there is a chance that your baby might not get HIV. For this reason, every pregnant woman who is HIV positive should be treated with medicine.

How would I know if I had the HIV virus?

The only way to know is to take the HIV antibody blood test.

What if my test is negative?

A negative test means that the antibody has not been found in your blood. But if you have had a recent exposure to HIV (within the last 6 months), then you should have the test now, have it again in 6 months, and again 6 months after that to be sure that you are really negative.

What if my test is positive?

A positive test means that the antibody is in your blood, and you are infected with the HIV virus. If this happens, you will be given special counseling, because you will have many important decisions to make regarding medications.

I'm married, and I don't have affairs. That means I'm safe, right?

Unfortunately that isn't true. You might have had sex several years ago (before you were married) with someone who was involved in bisexual sex or sex with an IV drug user. You might not have known about that, but you could be at risk. Also, your husband or current partner could have a sexual history you don't know about. A previous partner of his could have infected him, and he doesn't even know it.

Should I take the HIV test?

If you are pregnant now or planning to become pregnant, consider taking the test, especially if any of the risk categories apply to you. Even if you feel fine, you could be infected and then pass it on to your baby. Ask your provider to advise you on this.

How can I protect myself from HIV infection?

If you are HIV negative, then from now on:

- Use condoms if you have several sexual partners
- Use condoms with any sexual partner who has risk factors for HIV
- Don't share needles (drug use, tattooing, skin piercing)
- Practice safer sex (no anal sex)

Flesch-Kincaid Reading Level: 6.7

Special Instructions _____

Phone number to call if you have questions: _____

Copyright © 2002 Lippincott Williams & Wilkins. Developed by MC Freda, EdD, RN, CHES, FAAN.

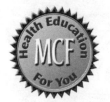
Health Education For You MCF

Woman's name: _____

Date: _____

Nurse's name: _____

Infección del Virus de Immunodeficiencia Humana y SIDA

Todos los proveedores de cuidado prenatal deberían de hablar con las mujeres embarazadas acerca del virus VIH. Probablemente usted tambien tenga preguntas sobre éste tema. Lea éste folleto y luego hable con su doctor, enfermera o comadrona.

¿Puede mi bebé nacer con el virus del SIDA?

Si usted está infectada con el virus VIH, existe el 50% de posibilidad que su bebé nazca infectado. Han habido estudios recientes que indican que si usted tiene el virus del VIH y que durante el embarazo ha estado tomando ciertas medicinas, existe la posibilidad de que su bebé no tenga el virus VIH. Es por este motivo que cualquier mujer embarazada que salga positiva en la prueba de HIV debe ser tratado con medicamentos.

¿Cómo se yo que tengo el virus VIH?

La única manera de saberlo es haciéndose la prueba de sangre anticuerpo VIH.

¿Qué pasaría si mis resultados salen negativos?

Una prueba con resultados negativos significaría que el anticuerpo no fué hallado en su sangre. Sin embargo, si usted ha estado expuesta al virus VIH (dentro de los últimos seis meses) entonces debería hacerse los exámenes ahora, repetirlos en 6 meses, y de nuevo en otros 6 meses, para así asegurar de que este libre de infección.

¿Qué pasaría si mis resultados salen positivos?

Una prueba con resultados positivos indicaría que el anticuerpo está presente en su sangre y que usted está infectada con el virus del VIH. Si esto sucediera, se le dará consejería especial ya que tendrá que tomar decisiones muy importantes sobre los medicamentos que tendrá que tomar.

Estoy casado y no tengo relaciones sexuales fuera del matrimonio. Estoy fuera de peligro ¿verdad?

Desafortunadamente esto no es verdad. Es posible que hace muchos años atrás (antes de que se casara) usted estubo involucrado en una relación bisexual o haya tenido sexo con una persona que se inyectaba drogas en las venas. Quizás usted desconocía esto, pero usted se expuso al peligro. Tambien puede ser posible que su esposo o pareja actual tenga una historia de relaciones sexuales que usted desconozca. Es posible que una antigua pareja lo haya infectado y ni siquiera se ha dado por enterado.

¿Debo hacerme el exámen del VIH?

Si usted está ahora embarazada ó planea salir embarazada, considere hacerse la prueba del SIDA, especialmente si corre alto riesgo. Y aunque usted se sienta bien de salud, podría estar infectada y luego transmitirlo a su bebé. Pídale a su proveedor que le aconseje sobre este tema.

¿Cómo me puedo proteger contra la infección del HIV?

- Si usted sale negativo en la prueba del SIDA, entonces de ahora en adelante:
- Use condones si tiene varias parejas sexuales.
- Use condones con cualquier pareja sexual que tenga altos riesgos de contraer el VIH
- No comparta agujas (para el uso de drogas, para hacerse tatuajes, perforaciones en la piel)
- Practique sexo sanamente (no sexo anal)

Special Instructions _____

Phone number to call if you have questions: _____

Copyright © 2002 Lippincott Williams & Wilkins. Developed by MC Freda, EdD, RN, CHES, FAAN.

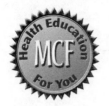
Health Education
MCF
For You

Woman's name: _____

Date: _____

Nurse's name: _____

Things You Need to Know About Chlamydia

Do you know what "chlamydia" (pronounced "kla-mid-ee-ah") infections are? They can be dangerous to your health, and you should learn as much as you can about how to protect yourself. This information sheet will help you learn about chlamydia infections. Please talk to your doctor, nurse, or midwife about this also.

What Is Chlamydia???

Chlamydia infections are a type of STD (sexually transmitted disease). You <u>only</u> get this infection when you have sex with a person who has chlamydia.

What Can Chlamydia Do To You???

Chlamydia is dangerous. It can cause both women and men to become sterile (not able to have children), and can cause women to have painful pelvic infections.

What Are the Symptoms of Chlamydia???

This is what makes chlamydia so different from other STDs. *In some women and men there are no symptoms*. In some women and men symptoms like pain when urinating or vaginal discharge <u>might</u> happen 7 to 35 days after having sex with an infected person, but *you probably cannot tell if you or your partner is infected.*

How Do You Know If You Have Chlamydia???

There is only one way to know, and that is a laboratory test.

What to Do If You Have Chlamydia

- Be sure to take all the antibiotics you are given. If you don't, then the infection will come right back.
- **Your sexual partner must be tested and take the medicine also.** If he doesn't take the medicine, he will give the infection back to you when you have sex.
- **Don't have sex until you have finished all the medicine.**
- Have another laboratory test done after the medicine is finished to see if the infection is gone.

Flesch-Kincaid Reading Level: 7.9

Special Instructions _____

_____

_____

Phone number to call if you have questions: _____

Copyright © 2002 Lippincott Williams & Wilkins. Developed by MC Freda, EdD, RN, CHES, FAAN.

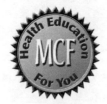

Woman's name: _____

Date: _____

Nurse's name: _____

Lo que usted debe saber sobre la Clamidia

¿Sabe usted lo que son las infecciones de Clamidia? Pueden ser peligrosas para su salud, y debe aprender lo más que pueda sobre como protejerse. Esta hoja de información le ayudará a aprender acerca de las infecciones de Clamidia. Por favor, hable con su doctor, enfermera, o partera acerca de esto.

¿¿¿Qué es la Clamidia???

Infecciones de Clamidia son un tipo de ETS (Enfermedades Transmitidas Sexualmente). Solamente le da esta infección si tiene relaciones sexuales con una person que tiene Clamidia.

¿¿¿Qué es lo que la Clamidia le puede hacer???

La Clamidia es peligrosa. Puede resultar en que ambos hombres y mujeres se vuelvan esteriles (no poder tener hijos), y puede causar infecciones pélvicas muy peligrosas en las mujeres.

¿¿¿Qué es lo que le puede occurir con la Clamidia???

Esto es lo que hace que la Clamidia sea tan diferente que las otras ETS's. **En algunos hombres y mujeres no hay síntomas.** En algunas mujeres y hombres síntomas como dolor al orinar o flujo vaginal pueden occurrir de 7 a 35 días depués de tener relaciones sexuales con una persona infectada pero usted **probablemente no prodrá distinguir si es que usted o su pareja está infectada.**

¿¿¿Cómo sabe si tiene Clamidia???

Hay solamente una manera de saber esto, y es con una prueba de laboratorio.

Que hacer si tiene Clamidia:

- Asegurarse de tomar todo los antibióticos que le den. Si no lo hace, entonces la infección regresará.
- **Su pareja sexual tendrá que hacerse la prueba y también deberá tomar el medicamento.** Si no toma el medicamento, le devolverá a usted la infección después de tener relaciones sexuales con usted.
- **No tenga relaciones sexuales hasta terminar toda la medicina.**
- Hagáse otra prueba después que se termine la medicina para ver si la infección ha desaparecido.

Special Instructions _____

_____

Phone number to call if you have questions: _____

Copyright © 2002 Lippincott Williams & Wilkins. Developed by MC Freda, EdD, RN, CHES, FAAN.

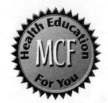

Woman's name: _____

Date: _____

Nurse's name: _____

Have You Heard About HPV?

What is HPV?

HPV is human papilloma virus. It used to be called "genital warts" or "venereal warts." HPV is a very common sexually transmitted disease. There may be as many as 24 million people infected with HPV in the United States.

Why should you be concerned about HPV?

HPV infections can lead to cancer of the cervix, so it is very important that you visit a doctor, nurse, or midwife if you think you have HPV.

What are the symptoms of HPV?

- You might have a heavy vaginal discharge that itches and hurts
- You might have pain when you have sexual intercourse
- You might have vaginal bleeding after sexual intercourse
- You might see warts on your vagina or on the skin around your vagina
- You might have warts inside your vagina or on your cervix (the mouth of your womb) that your doctor, nurse, or midwife can see when you are examined
- You might have no symptoms at all, but maybe your Pap test was abnormal

What should you do if you have HPV?

If your doctor, nurse, or midwife tells you that you have HPV, you need to do several things:

- Tell your sexual partners about your diagnosis. HPV is very contagious, so your partner or partners need to see a doctor also.
- HPV cannot be cured. It can only be treated so the symptoms are not as bad. This means that you must always use a condom for sex—always—or else you will give this disease to your partner.
- You need to use the medicine your provider gives you, exactly as prescribed.
- You will probably need to have a Pap test every 6 months, to watch for cancer of the cervix.

Flesch-Kincaid Reading Level: 5.4

Special Instructions _____

_____

_____

Phone number to call if you have questions: _____

Copyright © 2002 Lippincott Williams & Wilkins. Developed by MC Freda, EdD, RN, CHES, FAAN.

Woman's name: _____

Date: _____

Nurse's name: _____

¿Ha escuchado usted sobre el Virus de Papiloma Humano (VPH)

¿Qué es el VPH?

El VPH es el Virus de Papiloma Humano. Antes se le llamaba "verrugas genitales", o " verrugas venéreas" El VPH es una enfermedad transmitida sexualmente muy común. En los Estados Unidos pueden haber tanto como veinte y cuatro millones de personas infectadas con el VPH.

¿Por qué le debe preocupar el VPH?

Las infecciones del VPH pueden conducir al cáncer del cervix , así que es muy importante de que visite a un doctor, enfermera o comadrona si cree que tiene el VPH.

¿Cuáles son los síntomas del VPH?

- Usted puede tener una fuerte descarga vaginal que le puede picar y doler
- Usted puede sentir dolor cuando tenga relaciones sexuales
- Usted puede sangrar por la vagina después de tener sexo
- Usted puede notar verrugas en su vagina o en la piel alrededor de su vagina.
- Algunas veces las verrugas pueden estar dentro de su vagina o en su cervix (la boca de su matriz)
- Algunas veces usted puede carecer de síntomas, pero luego su Examen del Papanicolaou puede salir anormal.

¿Qué debe usted hacer si tiene el VPH?

Sí su doctor, enfermera o comadrona le informan de que usted tiene el VPH, existen varias cosas que usted debe de hacer:

- Informales a sus parejas sexuales acerca de su diagnóstico. El VPH es muy contagioso así que su pareja o parejas también necesitaran ver un doctor.
- El VPH no se puede curar. Solamente se puede tratar para que los síntomas no sean tan malos. Esto quiere decir de que usted debe siempre usar condones en sus relaciones sexuales o de lo contrario usted le transmitirá la enfermedad a su pareja.
- Usted debe tomar la medicina que le dió su doctor exactamente tal como se la recetó
- Probablemente usted necesitará hacerse la prueba de Papanicolau cada seis meses para vigilar el desarrollo del cáncer al cervix.

Special Instructions _____

_____

Phone number to call if you have questions: _____

Copyright © 2002 Lippincott Williams & Wilkins. Developed by MC Freda, EdD, RN, CHES, FAAN.

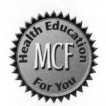

Woman's name: _____
Date: _____
Nurse's name: _____

Some Community Resources

AIDS Information Hotline   (410)342-2742
www.critpath.org/aric/index

Alcoholism Help   check local phone book
http://alcoholism.about.com/
http://www.aa.org

Breast-feeding Support   (800) 525-3243
(La Leche International)
http://www.laleche.org

National Child Abuse Hotline   (800) 4 A Child
                                                (800) 422-4453

Domestic Violence Hotline   (800) 799-SAFE
                                                (800) 799-7233

Safe Horizons (domestic violence help)   (800) 621-HOPE
www.dvsheltertour.org   (800) 621-4673

Substance Use Hotline   (800) 454-8966
http://substanceabuse.about.com/health/substanceabuse

Pregnancy Loss Resources
  RTS Bereavement Services   (608) 785-0530
  Compassionate Friends   (708) 990-0010
  http://www.compassionatefriends.org

Doulas of North America   (801) 756-7331
http://www.dona.com

Lamaze International   (800) 368-4404
http://www.lamaze.org

March of Dimes   (888) MODIMES
http://www.modimes.org   (888) 663-4637

Special Instructions _____

_____

_____

Phone number to call if you have questions: _____

Copyright © 2002 Lippincott Williams & Wilkins. Developed by MC Freda, EdD, RN, CHES, FAAN.

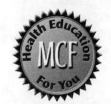

Woman's name: _____
Date: _____
Nurse's name: _____

Guía Telefónica Para La Comunidad

Información sobre el SIDA   (410) 342-2742
www.critpath.org/aric/index

Ayuda contra el Alcoholismo
http://alcoholism.about.com/
http://www.aa.org

Apoyo para Amamantar
(La Leche Internacional)
http://www.laleche.org   (800) 525-3243

Línea caliente contra el Abuso Infantil   (800) 4 A Child
                                                                (800) 422-4453

Línea caliente contra la Violencia Doméstica   (800) 799-SAFE
                                                                (800) 799-7233

Horizontes Seguros (ayuda contra la violencia doméstica)   (800) 621-HOPE
www.dvsheltertour.org   (800) 621-4673

Línea caliente contra el abuso de sustancias   (800) 454-8966
http://substanceabuse.about.com/health/substanceabuse

Pérdida del embarazo
  Amigos Compasivos   (608) 785-0530
  Servicios de Duelo   (708) 990-0010
  http://www.compassionatefriends.org

Doulas de NorteAmerica   (801) 756-7331
http://www.dona.com

Lamaze Internacional
http://www.lamaze.org   (800) 368-4404

March of Dimes   (888) MODIMES
http://www.modimes.org   (888) 663-4367

Special Instructions _____

_____

_____

Phone number to call if you have questions: _____

Copyright © 2002 Lippincott Williams & Wilkins. Developed by MC Freda, EdD, RN, CHES, FAAN.

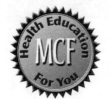

Woman's name: _____

Date: _____

Nurse's name: _____

Breast-Feeding or Bottle-Feeding? How Do I Decide?

Whatever decision you make about feeding your newborn baby will be the right one for you and your baby. Babies grow and are healthy on both breast-feeding and bottle-feeding. There are many things for you to think about in deciding whether to breast-feed or to bottle-feed. You should start to think about how you and your partner feel about this important topic so that you know what you want to do by the time your baby is born. Perhaps some of the issues discussed below will help you to decide.

Breast-feeding	Bottle-feeding
Breast milk has the correct amount of nutrients for the baby's growth and development	The baby's father can be involved in feeding the baby
	No diet restrictions for the woman
Breast milk protects babies from some illnesses	Women who must be away from their babies for periods of time will not have to worry about pumping their breasts and keeping the milk cold
Babies digest breast milk easily, and rarely have diarrhea or constipation	
Very few babies are ever allergic to breast milk	Women who return to work might feel that bottle-feeding will fit into their schedules more easily
Breast-feeding doesn't cost any money	Some women are concerned that breast-feeding their babies in public would be uncomfortable for them
Breast-feeding helps shrink the uterus back to size quickly	

You and your partner should discuss all these issues with your health care providers (including your baby's doctor or nurse practitioner) and read more about this. If you think that you want to breast-feed, give yourself several weeks of breast-feeding (probably 6 weeks is necessary) to decide how you, your partner, and your baby are doing.

Flesch-Kincaid Reading Level:6.8

Special Instructions _____

_____

Phone number to call if you have questions: _____

Copyright © 2002 Lippincott Williams & Wilkins. Developed by MC Freda, EdD, RN, CHES, FAAN.

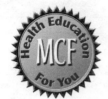

Woman's name: _____

Date: _____

Nurse's name: _____

¿¿¿El Pecho O La Botella????
¿¿¿Cómo Decido????

Cualquier decisión que tome acerca de la alimentación de su bebé será la correcta para usted y su bebé. Los niños crecen y son saludables con ambas formas de alimentacion, botella o pecho. Hay muchas cosas en que pensar acerca de dar el pecho o la botella. Debe comenzar a pensar acerca de como usted y su pareja se siente sobre este tema importante para que sepa lo que va a hacer al momento que su bebé nazca. Posiblemente, algunas de las siguientes sugerencias le ayudarán a decidir.

El pecho	La botella
La leche de pecho tiene la cantidad correcta de nutrientes para el crecimiento y desarollo del bebé	El padre del bebé puede participar en la alimentacion
	No hay dieta para la mujer
La leche de pecho proteje los bebés de algunas enfermedades	Las mujeres que tienen que separarse temporalmente de su bebé no tienen que extraerse la leche y mantenerla fría
Los bebés digieren mejor la leche de pecho y raramente les da diarrea o estreñimiento	
Muy pocos niños son alérgicos a la leche de pecho	Las mujeres que regresan al trabajo encuentran más favorable dar la botella
La alimentación del pecho no es costosa	Algunas mujeres se sienten incómodas dando el pecho al bebé en público
Dar el pecho le ayuda a que el útero se normalize más rápido	

Usted y su pareja deben discutir todos estos temas con su proveedor de salud (incluyendo el doctor del bebé o enfermera), y lea más sobre esto. Si quiere dar el pecho, permita algunas semanas (quizás 6 semanas) para decidir como su pareja y su bebé se sienten.

Special Instructions _____

_____

_____

Phone number to call if you have questions: _____

Copyright © 2002 Lippincott Williams & Wilkins. Developed by MC Freda, EdD, RN, CHES, FAAN.

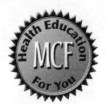

Woman's name: _____

Date: _____

Nurse's name: _____

Sex During Pregnancy

I'm worried about having sex during pregnancy. Can it hurt the baby?

Sex during pregnancy does not hurt the baby. There are only a few exceptions to this rule. If your water has broken, you should not have sex or put anything in your vagina. The bag of waters protects the baby from infection. Once it has broken the baby can become infected. The only other time it might be a bad idea to have sex is if you feel a lot of uterine contractions after you have sex. Some doctors, nurses, or midwives might suggest that you stop having sex until the risk of preterm labor is gone (around 36 weeks of pregnancy).

I don't really want to have sex now. Is there something wrong with me?

Some women have a change in their desire for sex during pregnancy. There is nothing wrong with you. You might be too nauseous or too uncomfortable to have sex right now, but you will feel like it again in the future. Talk to your partner about this and be honest about how you are feeling. Some pregnant women might want to have sex more often than before. That's normal, too.

Are there sexual things we shouldn't do during pregnancy?

Anal sex is not safe sex due to the high risk of bleeding and getting diseases. Anal sex is a bad idea during pregnancy as well. Also, your partner should not blow into your vagina during oral sex. This can cause air bubbles to go into blood vessels in the uterus and can be dangerous to the baby and to you.

What about sex at the end of pregnancy when I'm so big?

If you feel well, there is no medical reason why you would have to stop having sex until your water breaks. Your larger uterus might make it difficult or uncomfortable to have the man on top. You can try different positions such as you being on top or you lying on your side. If intercourse is uncomfortable, there are other sexual things you and your partner can do to pleasure each other, such as using your hands. Oral sex is also an option. As long as the sex is loving and is the choice of both partners, you will find ways to be happy and comfortable.

If you don't feel well enough right now to have sex, explain that to your partner. People who love each other understand that sex is only appropriate when both partners want it. Never allow anyone to force you to have sex against your will.

Flesch-Kincaid Reading Level: 6.4

Special Instructions _____

Phone number to call if you have questions: _____

Copyright © 2002 Lippincott Williams & Wilkins. Developed by MC Freda, EdD, RN, CHES, FAAN.

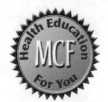

Woman's name: _____

Date: _____

Nurse's name: _____

Sexo durante el Embarazo

Me preocupa tener sexo durante el embarazo. ¿Puedo dañar al bebé?

Sexo durante el embarazo no daña al bebé. Sin embargo, hay unas cuantas excepciones a ésta regla. No deberías tener sexo si la fuente de agua se ha roto, o insertar algo dentro de vagina. La bolsa de agua proteje al bebé de infecciones. Una vez rota la bolsa, el bebé puede infectarse. Hay otra situación donde no es conveniente tener sexo y es cuando sientes muchas contracciones uterinas después de tener relaciones íntimas. Algunos doctores, enfermeras o comadronas podrían sugerirte que te abstengas de tener relaciones hasta que el riesgo de un parto prematuro pase (alrededor de la 36va semana de embarazo)

No tengo deseo de tener relaciones sexuales. ¿Hay algo malo conmigo?

Algunas mujeres experimentan cambios en el deseo sexual durante el embarazo. No hay nada de malo en ésto. Pueda ser que te sientas con muchas náuseas o muy incómoda como para tener relaciones, pero no te preocupes porque volverás a sentir deseo otra vez en el futuro. Habla con tu pareja sobre ésto y sé lo más honesta posible sobre lo que sientes. Algunas mujeres embarazadas sienten más deseo de tener relaciones que antes de quedar embarazadas. Esto tambien es normal.

¿Hay algun tipo de acto sexual que no debamos hacer durante el embarazo?

No es recomendable tener sexo anal ya que existe la posibilidad de sangramiento y contraer otras enfermedades. Sexo anal es una mala idea durante el embarazo. Tambien tu pareja no debe de soplar dentro de tu vagina durante sexo oral. Esto causa burbujas de aire que van dentro de los capilares sanguíneos en el útero y puede ser muy peligroso para tí y tu bebé.

¿Y qué puedo hacer hacia el final del embarazo cuando estoy muy grande y pesada?

Si te sientes bien, no hay ninguna razón médica por la cual no deberías de tener sexo, a menos que se te rompa la fuente de agua. Pueder se un poco difícil o íncomodo tener un hombre encima de tí cuando tu útero ha crecido tanto. Puedes tratar otras posiciones, como estar tu arriba o acostarte de lado. Si las relaciones íntimas son incómodas, existen otras cosas sexuales que tu y tu pareja podrían hacer para sentir placer, como usar las manos. Sexo oral tambien es una opción. Siempre y cuando el sexo es tierno y amoroso y es lo que han escogido ambas parejas, encontrarás formas de sentirte feliz y cómoda.

Si no te sientes lo suficientemente bien como para tener sexo por el momento, explícaselo a tu pareja. Las personas que se aman comprenden que el sexo es sólo apropiado cuando ambos lo desean. Nunca permitas que nadie te force a tener sexo contra tu voluntad.

Special Instructions _____

_____

Phone number to call if you have questions: _____

Copyright © 2002 Lippincott Williams & Wilkins. Developed by MC Freda, EdD, RN, CHES, FAAN.

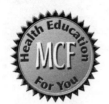

What Is a Doula?

Maybe you never heard the word "doula" (pronounced "doo-lah"). Many people haven't. But now that you're pregnant, you might want to know about doulas. A doula is a person who believes that birth is a normal process and has been specially trained to provide support to you during labor. Doulas are not nurses or doctors. They are just regular people, but they have learned how to help you be most comfortable without drugs during labor. Many women enjoy having a doula with them in labor, for the doula is only working for you and with you. She has no one else to care for and will stay with you when you are in labor and giving birth. She has been trained in helping laboring women breathe properly and relax during labor and for helping women find the most comfortable positions for labor and for giving birth. Some doulas have also been trained in massage for women in labor. A doula is not a midwife and will not actually deliver your baby. She will focus on giving you support.

Why would you want a doula?

- Some women have no other support person to be with them in labor
- Some women feel that a doula will help them get through their labor without medications
- Not all husbands or partners know very much about how to be supportive during labor, and some don't really want to participate in that way
- There is some research showing that women who have doulas are very satisfied with their birth experiences

How do you find a doula?

There is an organization called Doulas of North America (DONA) that certifies qualified doulas. Its Website is: www.dona.com. DONA will give you names of doulas in your area.

Be sure to ask any doula you interview about her training, her philosophy of birthing, her fees, what hospitals or birthing centers she works with, and if there is a backup doula in case she is with another woman when you go into labor.

Be sure to discuss this with your doctor, midwife, or nurse. You need to know how he or she feels about doulas if you are considering using one. Some hospitals do not allow doulas, and you need to know about this if you want one.

Flesch-Kincaid Reading Level: 7.4

Special Instructions _____

_____

Phone number to call if you have questions: _____

Copyright © 2002 Lippincott Williams & Wilkins. Developed by MC Freda, EdD, RN, CHES, FAAN.

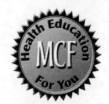

Woman's name: _____

Date: _____

Nurse's name: _____

¿Qué es una Doula?

Quizás nunca has escuchado la palabra "doula". Muchas personas nunca lo han escuchado. Pero ahora que estás embarazada, deberías de informarte sobre lo que son las doulas. Una doula es una persona que piensa que el nacimiento es un proceso natural, y han sido especialmente entrenadas para proveer soporte mientras nace el bebé. Doulas no son enfermeras ó doctores. Estas son personas communes que han aprendido como ayudar a las personas a sentirse más cómoda sin usar drogas durante el parto. Muchas mujeres agradecen el poder tener un doula con ellas durante el parto, porque la doula no sólo trabaja para tí sino contigo también. Ella no tiene nadie más quien cuidar y permanecerá contigo durante el parto y el nacimiento. Ella ha sido entrenada en ayudar a mujeres parturientas a respirar en la forma correcta y a relajarse durante el parto, y ayudarles a encontrar la major posición para el parto y el nacimiento del bebé. Algunas doulas han sido entrenadas para dar masajes a las mujeres parturientas. Ella no es una comadrona, ella no va a ayudar con el nacimineto del bebé. Ella se enfocará en darte soporte moral.

¿Porqué querías tener una doula?

- Algunas mujeres no tienen a nadie que las soporten moralmente.
- Algunas mujeres sienten que una doula las ayudarán a dar a luz sin utilizar ningún medicamento.
- No todos los esposos o parejas saben como ser cooperativos durante el parto, y algunos en realidad no quieren participar en ésa forma.
- Existen algunos estudios que demuestran que las mujeres que tienen doulas están muy satisfechas con sus experiencias durante el nacimiento del bebé.

¿Cómo encontrarás una doula?

Existe una organización llamada Doulas de Norte America (DONA) el cual certifica doulas calificadas. Su página del internet es: www.dona.com DONA te dará los nombres de las doulas en tu área.

Asegúrate de preguntar a la doula que estás entrevistando, cual es su filosofía sobre el nacimiento, sus honorarios, con cual hospital o centro de maternidad trabaja, y si hay una doula de emergencia en caso que la otra doula esté con otra mujer cuando tu estés en parto.

Asegúrate de discutir esto con tu doctor, comadrona o enfermera. Necesitas saber cuales son sus opinions sobre las doulas ,si estás considerando usar de sus servicios. Algunos hospitales no permiten doulas y debes estar prevenida en caso que vayas a usar sus servicios

Special Instructions _____

_____

Phone number to call if you have questions: _____

Copyright © 2002 Lippincott Williams & Wilkins. Developed by MC Freda, EdD, RN, CHES, FAAN.

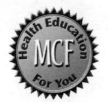

Woman's name: _____

Date: _____

Nurse's name: _____

The Ultrasound Test

What Is the Ultrasound?

Ultrasound is also called "sonogram." Your doctor, midwife, or nurse can look into your uterus and see your baby and the placenta (afterbirth) using ultrasound. With special training, your provider can then see how the baby is growing. Sometime he or she can even see whether the baby is a girl or a boy. You don't have to do anything special to get ready for this test when you are pregnant. It does not hurt. If your provider has the equipment, you might be given a picture of the baby to take home after the ultrasound.

How Is the Ultrasound Done?

There are two ways of doing this test. For the abdominal ultrasound, you lie on a table, and the provider places a small amount of gel on a disk and then moves it around on your abdomen. A picture of what is inside your uterus appears on a television screen. The provider will explain what you are seeing (sometimes it's hard to understand what you're seeing without that help).

The second way of doing an ultrasound is through the vagina. It is just like having a vaginal examination. You lie on your back with your knees apart, and the provider puts an instrument in your vagina. Then you look at the screen together and see the pictures of the baby and the placenta.

When Should an Ultrasound Be Done?

Ultrasounds are usually done a few times in each pregnancy. Once in the beginning of pregnancy to be sure you are pregnant. Once again at about 20 weeks of pregnancy to be sure that the baby is growing properly. Then whenever the provider thinks it's important to see the baby or the placenta he or she might do it again. There is no known harm to the baby or the mother from having ultrasounds. They do cost money, and therefore insurance companies will usually only pay for ultrasounds that your provider thinks are really necessary.

Flesch-Kincaid Reading Level: 7.1

Special Instructions _____

_____

_____

_____

Phone number to call if you have questions: _____

Copyright © 2002 Lippincott Williams & Wilkins. Developed by MC Freda, EdD, RN, CHES, FAAN.

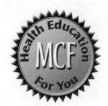

Woman's name: _____

Date: _____

Nurse's name: _____

La Prueba del Ultrasonido

¿Qué es el Ultrasonido?

Al ultrasonido también se le llama "sonograma". Su doctor , comadrona o enfermera pueden mirar dentro de su útero y mirar a su bebé y a la placenta mediante el uso de una máquina de ultrasonido. Con entrenamiento especial, su doctor puede ver como su bebé se está desarrollando. Algunas veces ellos pueden ver el sexo del bebé. Usted no tiene que hacer nada en especial para estar lista para esta prueba cuando esté embarazada. No le produce dolor. Inclusive si su proveedor tiene el equipo necesario usted se podrá llevar una foto del bebé después de la prueba de ultrasonido.

¿Cómo se efectua el Ultrasonido?

Hay dos maneras de hacer esta prueba. Para el ultrasonido abdominal, usted se acuesta sobre una mesa, y el doctor coloca una pequeña cantidad de gel sobre un disco el cual luego lo pasa alrededor de su abdomen. Luego una foto de lo que esta dentro de su útero aparecerá en una pantalla de televisión. El doctor le irá explicando lo que va viendo(algunas veces es dificíl de comprender lo que uno está viendo sin la ayuda del doctor).

La segunda manera de realizar el ultrasonido es a través de la vagina. Es tal como si le estuviesen haciendo un exámen vaginal. Se acuesta sobre su espalda con las rodillas aparte y el doctor le introduce un aparato en su vagina. Luego juntos ven en la pantalla las fotos del bebé y la placenta.

¿Cuándo se debe realizar una prueba de Ultrasonido?

Durante el embarazo algunas mujeres no se someten al sonograma mientras que otras sí lo hacen. Cuando las pruebas son hechas generalmente se hacen al comienzo del embarazo para asegurarse de que estan embarazadas. Se hace una vez más; alrededor de las 20 semanas de embarazo para asegurase de que el bebé esté desarrollándose normalmente. Y luego en cualquier momento en que el doctor considere importante ver al bebé o la placenta, se le hará la prueba de nuevo. No se conoce de ningún daño causado a la mamá o bebé por someterse a la prueba del sonograma. En vista de que los sonogramas cuestan dinero las compañías de seguro solo pagarán por aquellas pruebas que los doctores consideren necesarias.

Special Instructions _____

_____

_____

Phone number to call if you have questions: _____

Copyright © 2002 Lippincott Williams & Wilkins. Developed by MC Freda, EdD, RN, CHES, FAAN.

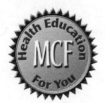

Woman's name: _____
Date: _____
Nurse's name: _____

The Biophysical Profile

What Is the Biophysical Profile?

This is a special test done when more information is needed about your baby's health. Not all providers can do a biophysical profile. They need special machines and special training to do it. Many times biophysical profiles are done in university hospitals.

How Is a Biophysical Profile Done?

The test is done using ultrasound (see previous handout on ultrasound). It does not hurt.

When Would a Biophysical Profile Be Ordered?

This would be ordered if your provider thinks the baby might need to be delivered soon. Five different things about the baby are measured: (1) body movements, (2) breathing movements, (3) muscle tone, (4) amount of amniotic fluid surrounding the baby, and (5) the way the baby's heart reacts to movement. A score is given for each area. Normal for each is scored as 2. The highest possible score for the biophysical profile is 10.

The score, along with other factors, will be used to help make some decisions about whether your baby is healthy enough to stay in your uterus or whether it would be better for your baby to be born sooner.

Be sure to ask your doctor, nurse, or midwife any questions you have about the biophysical profile.

Flesch-Kincaid Reading Level: 7.8

Special Instructions _____

_____

_____

_____

_____

_____

Phone number to call if you have questions: _____

Copyright © 2002 Lippincott Williams & Wilkins. Developed by MC Freda, EdD, RN, CHES, FAAN.

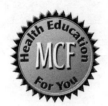

Woman's name: _____

Date: _____

Nurse's name: _____

El Perfil Biofísico

¿Qué es el Perfil Biofísico?

Este es un procedimiento especial requerido cuando se necesita más información sobre la salud del bebé. No todos los doctores realizan un perfil biofísico. Ellos necesitan máquinas especiales y un entrenamiento especial para realizarlo. Muchas veces los perfiles biofísicos se hacen en las universidades de los hospitales o en los centros médicos.

¿Cómo se realiza el Perfil Biofísico?

La prueba se hace usando ultrasonido (vea el manual anterior sobre ultrasonido). No es doloroso.

¿Cuándo se requiere de un Perfil Biofísico?

Esto es ordenado cuando el doctor piensa que el bebé debe de nacer antes de tiempo. Hay cinco diferentes tipos de medidas en que el bebé es evaluado (1) los movimientos del cuerpo, (2) los movimientos respiratorios, (3) el tono muscular, (4) el líquido amniótico alrededor del bebé, y (5) la forma en que el corazón del bebé reacciona a los movimientos. Cierto puntaje es asignado a cada sección. Un puntaje de 2 es asignado a cada lectura normal; 10 es el puntaje más alto para un perfil biofísico.

El puntaje, junto con otros factores, será utilizado para decidir si el bebé está lo suficientemente sano como para permanecer en el útero o si sería mejor hacer de que el bebé nazca mucho antes.

Asegúrese de preguntarle a su doctor, enfermera o comadrona cualquier interrogante que tenga sobre el perfil biofísico.

Special Instructions _____

_____

_____

_____

_____

_____

Phone number to call if you have questions: _____

Copyright © 2002 Lippincott Williams & Wilkins. Developed by MC Freda, EdD, RN, CHES, FAAN.

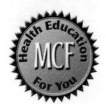

Woman's name: _____

Date: _____

Nurse's name: _____

Nonstress Tests

What Is a Nonstress Test?

This test has a strange name—"non stress test". The "stress" has nothing to do with how "stressed" you feel. The stress has to do with your uterus. Non-stress means that your providers want to find out how your baby is doing when there is no stress (really meaning contractions) happening to your uterus. The providers are trying to predict how healthy your baby is and how well your baby will react to the stress of labor. If a baby seems healthy when there is no stress on the uterus, your provider hopes that the baby will remain healthy when the stress of labor begins. A nonstress test is usually done to be sure your baby's heart rate pattern is normal.

When Would a Nonstress Test Be Ordered?

This test is usually ordered when you have a risk factor that might make your provider concerned about the baby's health during labor. For instance, women who have sicknesses in pregnancy (like diabetes or high blood pressure) or women whose pregnancy has passed their due date (called "Post Dates") might have nonstress tests. Other reasons for a nonstress test could be if a baby has been growing too slowly ("intrauterine growth restriction") or if it seems that there is not enough fluid around the baby.

How Is a Nonstress Test Done?

This test does not hurt. It might be done in the doctor's, nurse's, or midwife's office, or it might be done at a special place in the hospital. It usually takes 20 to 30 minutes. You usually sit in a comfortable chair and a nurse or other provider puts 2 elastic belts around your abdomen. They are attached to a fetal monitor. They record the baby's heartbeat and your uterine contractions, if you have any. Each time you feel the baby move, you either push a button or tell the provider. This makes a mark on the monitor paper. If the baby's heartbeat always goes up when he or she moves, then the test is over. If it doesn't, then they might continue the test longer or notify your doctor, nurse, or midwife who will decide what to do next.

Be sure to ask your doctor, nurse, or midwife if you have questions about this test.

Flesch-Kincaid Reading Level: 6.6

Special Instructions _____

_____

_____

Phone number to call if you have questions: _____

Copyright © 2002 Lippincott Williams & Wilkins. Developed by MC Freda, EdD, RN, CHES, FAAN.

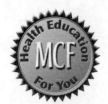

Woman's name: _____

Date: _____

Nurse's name: _____

Pruebas de No-Estrés

¿Qué es una prueba de No-Estrés?

Esta prueba tiene un nombre raro- "prueba de no estrés". El estrés no tiene nada que ver con lo que cuán tensionado usted se siente. Ni es tampoco como las pruebas que se hacen para el corazón. Este estrés está relacionado con su útero. No-Estrés significa que sus doctores quieren averiguar como le vá a su bebé cuando no hay estrés (contracciones) ocurriendo en su útero. Lo que sus doctores tratan de predecir es cuán saludable está su bebé y que bien reaccionará al estrés causado por el parto. Si el bebé se vé saludable cuando no hay estrés en el útero, entonces hay mayores posibilidades de que su bebé se mantenga saludable cuando empieze el estrés del parto. Generalmente, la prueba de no estrés se realiza para asegurarse de que el patrón de los latidos del corazón de su bebé esté normal.

¿Cuándo se debería de ordenar una prueba de No Estrés?

Generalmente ésta prueba se ordena cuando usted tiene un factor de riesgo que pudiese afectar la salud del bebé durante el parto. Por ejemplo, mujeres que están enfermas durante el embarazo (tal como diabetes o presión alta), o mujeres que se hayan pasado la fecha de dar a luz (llamada Post-Fecha o vencida) deberían de hacerse la prueba de no estrés. Otras razones para hacerse la prueba del no estrés sería por el lento crecimiento del bebé(restricción de crecimiento intrauterino) o si pareciera de que no hubiese demasiada cantidad de líquido alrededor del bebé.

¿Cómo se efectua la prueba del No-Estrés?

Esta prueba no causa dolor. Se puede hacer en la oficina del doctor, enfermera o comadrona o en algún lugar del hospital. Generalmente se toma de 20 a 30 minutos. Usualmente se sienta en un sillón cómodo y una enfermera u otro doctor le colocan 2 correas elásticas alrededor de su abdomen. Ellas están conectadas a un monitor fetal. Ellos registran los latidos el corazón del bebé y las contracciones de su útero; si tuviese alguna. Cada vez que usted siente que su bebé se mueve usted puede apretar un botón o avisarle a su doctor. Esto marcará la cinta del monitor. Si los latidos del corazón del bebé siempre señalan hacia arriba cuando el bebé sé mueve entonces la prueba se da por terminada.De lo contrario, ellos tendrán que continuar con la prueba por más tiempo o avisarle a su doctor, enfermera o comadrona quienes decidirán que hacer después.

Asegúrese de preguntarle a su doctor , enfermera o comadrona cualquier duda que tenga sobre esta prueba.

Special Instructions _____

_____

Phone number to call if you have questions: _____

Copyright © 2002 Lippincott Williams & Wilkins. Developed by MC Freda, EdD, RN, CHES, FAAN.

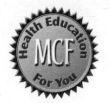

Woman's name: _____

Date: _____

Nurse's name: _____

Should You Take Childbirth Classes?

Most hospitals and birthing centers offer childbirth classes. Childbirth classes are usually offered by nurses or others who are called certified childbirth educators. The classes are usually offered one evening a week for about 6 weeks. Some instructors offer the classes on weekends or during the day as well.

Should you take childbirth education classes?

Yes, it is a good idea to take these classes. Most of the time you can go with a support person.

What happens in the classes?

Both you and your support person will learn about pregnancy and labor. You will also learn what to expect at your hospital or birthing center and how to cope with any problems or discomforts you have while pregnant. Many childbirth classes also show movies about labor and birth and get you ready for participating in your birth experience. Most people who take the classes find them very helpful. You can ask as many questions as you like. You will also probably be given a tour of the hospital or birthing center where you will give birth.

Will the classes cost money?

Most childbirth education classes cost money. The amount of money depends on where you live. Some free clinics offer the classes for free.

How can you find out about classes in your area?

You should ask your doctor, nurse, or midwife about childbirth education classes given where you live. You should also ask your friends who have taken classes in the past who they went to and whether they liked the classes.

Flesch-Kincaid Reading Level:6.4

Special Instructions _____

_____

_____

_____

_____

Phone number to call if you have questions: _____

Copyright © 2002 Lippincott Williams & Wilkins. Developed by MC Freda, EdD, RN, CHES, FAAN.

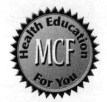

Woman's name: _____

Date: _____

Nurse's name: _____

¿Debe usted Tomar Clases de Parto?

La mayoría de los hospitales y maternidades ofrecen clases de parto. Generalmente , las clases de parto son ofrecidas por enfermeras u otras llamadas Instructores de Parto. Las clases son generalmente ofrecidas una noche a la semana por alrededor de seis semanas. Algunos instructores ofrecen las clases los fines de semana o también durante el día.

¿Debe usted tomar clases de educación natal?

Sí, es una buena idea tomar éstas clases. La mayoría de las veces usted puede ir acompañada con una persona de apoyo.

¿Qué ocurre en las clases?

Ambos, usted y su persona de apoyo aprenderan sobre el embarazo y el parto. Usted aprenderá lo que debe esperar de su hospital o maternidad, y como enfrentarse a cualquier problemas o molestias que tenga mientras está embarazada. En muchas clases de parto también le muestran películas sobre el nacimiento y el parto y la preparán para que participe en su experiencia del alumbramiento. La mayoría de las personas que toman las clases, las encuentran muy útiles. Usted puede hacer todas las preguntas que quiera. Probablemente también le daran un recorrido del hospital o centro de maternidad donde usted va a dar a luz.

¿Tendré que pagar por las clases?

Hay que pagar por la mayoría de las clases de parto. La cantidad de dinero depende de la zona donde vive. Algunas clínicas gratuitas ofrecen clases gratis.

¿Cómo puede averiguar sobre las clases en su comunidad?

Usted debe preguntarle a su doctor, enfermera o comadrona sobre las clases de educación natal ofrecidas en su comunidad.Usted también debe de preguntarle a sus amistades que en el pasado hayan tomado clases, a donde quien acudieron y si disfrutaron de las clases.

Special Instructions _____

_____

_____

_____

Phone number to call if you have questions: _____

Copyright © 2002 Lippincott Williams & Wilkins. Developed by MC Freda, EdD, RN, CHES, FAAN.

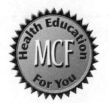
Your Blood Type and Rh Disease

Do you know your blood type? Do you know the blood type of the baby's father? It's important that you know this. During your first prenatal visit your doctor, nurse, or mid-wife did a blood test to find out your blood type. You should ask what he or she found. Your blood type will be a letter and then the word "positive" or the word "negative." You could be type A positive, type B positive, type AB positive, or type O positive. Or you could be type A negative, type B negative, type AB negative, or type O negative. If you are "positive," that means you have something in your blood called the Rh factor (you are "positive"). If you are "negative," that means you do not have the Rh factor in your blood (you are "negative"). Having the Rh factor in your blood is not a disease. Everyone is either Rh positive or Rh negative.

What Is Rh Disease?

If you are a woman who is Rh negative, and the father of your baby is Rh positive, you need to know about Rh disease. It is a special problem in pregnancy that can make the unborn baby very sick and sometimes die. When an Rh-negative woman has a baby with an Rh-positive man, the baby can be either Rh negative like the mother or Rh positive like the father. **This disease only happens when the woman is Rh negative, the man is Rh positive, and the baby is Rh positive like the father. If the baby is Rh negative like the mother, there is no problem.** It is now possible to prevent this disease by taking a special medicine, so it is very important that you know your blood type **and** the blood type of the baby's father.

How Does Rh Disease Happen?

- During the pregnancy or at the time of birth, the baby's blood cells mix in with the mother's. If the baby is Rh positive, like the father, the mother's blood tries to fight off the baby's Rh-positive factor. It's almost like the mother is allergic to the baby. The mother's blood develops antibodies to kill the Rh-positive factor. If the baby is Rh negative, like the mother, there is no problem and the mother's body never develops the antibodies.
- If the woman becomes pregnant with another Rh-positive baby, her body's immune system attacks the baby's blood to fight it off with the antibodies. This can make this baby extremely sick and even die.

How Can Rh Disease Be Prevented?

There is a drug that can be given to an Rh-negative mother during pregnancy and after she gives birth to an Rh-positive baby. It is a shot, called RhoGAM. This drug stops the mother's blood from developing those antibodies, which can hurt an Rh-positive baby. **It is important that an Rh-negative mother get this shot at the end of any pregnancy, even a miscarriage.** This will prevent the problem from happening in the next pregnancy.

You should talk to your doctor, nurse, or midwife about this if you are Rh negative.

Flesch-Kincaid Reading Level: 7.0

Special Instructions _____

_____

Phone number to call if you have questions: _____

Copyright © 2002 Lippincott Williams & Wilkins. Developed by MC Freda, EdD, RN, CHES, FAAN.

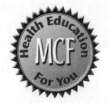

Woman's name: _____
Date: _____
Nurse's name: _____

Su Tipo de Sangre y la Enfermedad Rh

¿Conoce usted su tipo de sangre? ¿Conoce usted el tipo de sangre del padre de su bebé?. Es importante que usted sepa ésto. Durante su primera visita prenatal su doctor, enfermera o comadrona le hicieron un exámen de sangre para averiguar su tipo de sangre. Usted debe de preguntar lo que encontraron. Su tipo de sangre consistirá de una letra seguido por la palabra "positivo" o la palabra "negativo". Usted podría ser Tipo A positivo, Tipo B positivo, Tipo AB positivo o Tipo O positivo. O usted podría ser Tipo A negativo, Tipo B negativo, Tipo AB negativo o Tipo O negativo. Sí usted es "positivo", ésto significa de que tiene algo en su sangre llamado el factor Rh (usted és "positivo"). Sí usted es negativo, ésto significa de que usted no tiene en su sangre el factor Rh (usted es "negativo"). El tener el factor Rh en su sangre no es tener una enfermedad. Cada persona es Rh positivo o Rh negativo.

¿Qué es la enfermedad Rh?

Sí usted es una mujer quién es Rh negativo, y el padre de su bebé es Rh positivo, usted necesita saber de algo llamado "Enfermedad Rh". Es un problema especial del embarazo el cuál puede enfermar severamente al bebé aún no nacido y algunas veces fallecer. Cuando una mujer Rh negativa tiene un bebé con un hombre Rh positivo, el bebé podría ser Rh negativo como la madre o Rh positivo como el padre. **Esta enfermedad solamente ocurre cuando la mujer es Rh negativo, el padre es Rh positivo y el bebé es Rh positivo como él. Si el bebé es Rh negativo como la madre entonces no hay problema**. Ahora es posible evitar ésta enfermedad tomando una medicina especial, así que es muy importante saber su tipo de sangre **y** el tipo de sangre del padre de su bebé.

¿Cómo ocurre la enfermedad del Rh?

- Durante el embarazo o al momento de dar a luz, las células sanguíneas del bebé se mezclan con las de la madre. Si el bebé es Rh positivo, como el padre, la sangre de la madre trata de rechazar el factor Rh positivo del bebé. Es casi como si la madre fuera alérgica al bebé. La sangre de la madre produce anticuerpos que matan el factor Rh positivo. Si el bebé es Rh negativo como la madre, no hay problema porque el cuerpo de la mamá nunca produce aquellos anticuerpos.
- Si la mujer sale embarazada con otro bebé Rh positivo, el sistema inmunológico de ella atacará la sangre del bebé para rechazar a los anticuerpos. Esto podría causar del que el bebé se enferme severamente y hasta morirse.

¿Cómo se puede prevenir la enfermedad del Rh?

Existe una droga que se le puede dar a una madre Rh negativo durante su embarazo y después ella dará a luz a un bebé Rh positivo. Es una inyección llamada RhoGAM. Esta droga impide de que la sangre de la madre produzca aquellos anticuerpos que pueden causar daño a un bebé Rh positivo. **Es importante de que una madre Rh negativo obtenga ésta inyección al final de su embarazo e inclusive al de un aborto**. Esto evitará de que el problema ocurra en el próximo embarazo.

Si usted es Rh negativo no deje de hablar con su doctor, enfermera o comadrona.

Special Instructions _____

Phone number to call if you have questions: _____

Copyright © 2002 Lippincott Williams & Wilkins. Developed by MC Freda, EdD, RN, CHES, FAAN.

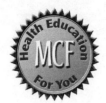

Woman's name: _____

Date: _____

Nurse's name: _____

What About Traveling During Pregnancy?

Life doesn't stop when you're pregnant. You still might want to travel for your job or on a planned vacation. What should you do?

Should you travel while you're pregnant?

It depends on a few factors.

- Most pregnancies are completely normal. In a normal pregnancy you can expect that everything will be fine, so traveling before your eighth month shouldn't be a problem.
- If you are having a high-risk pregnancy, traveling is not such a good idea. If you are having a multiple birth or if you have diabetes or some other sickness during pregnancy, it's better to be closer to your doctor and your hospital. If you travel far from home and become sick or go into premature labor, you'd have to find new doctors to take care of you.

If you travel, what can you do to be safe?

- You should not travel far from home after your eighth month of pregnancy. If you have to travel many hours from home, ask your doctor, nurse, or midwife for a copy of your medical record. You can carry it with you in case you need to see a provider away from home.
- If you must travel, choose a place that has good medical care available. A remote romantic island might sound like a nice vacation, but if you need medical care and there is no doctor or hospital, you could have a problem.
- If you travel on an airplane, be sure to get up and move around every 30 minutes. It's important to exercise your legs so you don't get blood clots in them.
- If you will be traveling in a car, stop every hour and get out and walk around to exercise your legs.
- Drinking enough fluids is important when you travel. Drink about 8 glasses of water each day.
- If you are traveling and you feel that something is not right with your pregnancy, call your provider and get advice about what to do. Don't just wait and hope it will go away.

Flesch-Kincaid Reading Level:6.1

Special Instructions _____

_____

_____

Phone number to call if you have questions: _____

Copyright © 2002 Lippincott Williams & Wilkins. Developed by MC Freda, EdD, RN, CHES, FAAN.

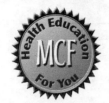

Woman's name: _____

Date: _____

Nurse's name: _____

¿Qué le parece viajar durante el embarazo?

La vida no se detiene por estar embarazada. Usted todavía desará viajar a su trabajo o irse de vacaciones. ¿Qué debería usted hacer?

¿Debe usted viajar mientras que está embarazada?

Ello depende de algunos factores.

- La mayoría de los embarazos son completamente normales. En un embarazo normal usted puede esperar de que todo salga bien. Así de que el viajar hasta el octavo més no presenta ningún problema.
- Si usted va a tener un embarazo con factores de alto riesgo, el viajar no sería una buena idea. Sí usted va a tener un nacimiento múltiple, o si tiene diabetes o alguna otra enfermedad mientras que esté embarazada, es mejor estar cerca a su doctor y a su hospital. Si usted viaja lejos de su casa y se enferma o tiene un parto prematuro tendría que encontrar nuevos doctores para que la atiendan.

¿Si viaja , qué puede usted hacer para sentirse segura?

- Usted no debe de viajar lejos de su casa después de su octavo més de embarazo.Si usted tiene que viajar a muchas horas fuera de su casa, pídale a su doctor, enfermera o comadrona una copia de su historial médico. Usted se lo puede llevar consigo en caso de que necesite ver a un doctor lejos de su casa.
- Si usted debe viajar, eliga un lugar que disponga de buenos servicios médicos. Una isla romántica y remota suena como unas vacaciones muy bonitas, pero si necesita atención médica y no hay un doctor o hospital al alcance, entonces usted podría tener un problema.
- Si usted viaja por avión, asegúrese de levantarse y moverse alrededor de cada treinta minutos. Es importante de que ejercite sus piernas de tal manera de que no se le formen coágulos de sangre.
- Si va a viajar por auto, pare cada treinta minutos, salga y camine alrededor para ejercitar sus piernas.
- Cuando viaje es importante que tome suficiente líquidos. Tome alrededor de ocho vasos de agua cada día.
- Si usted está viajando y siente que algo no anda bien con su embarazo, llame a su doctor y pregúntele que hacer. No se quede sin hacer nada y esperar a que la situación desaparezca.

Special Instructions _____

_____

_____

Phone number to call if you have questions: _____

Copyright © 2002 Lippincott Williams & Wilkins. Developed by MC Freda, EdD, RN, CHES, FAAN.

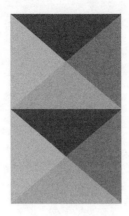

chapter 10

Intrapartum Care

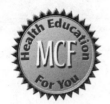

Woman's name: _____

Date: _____

Nurse's name: _____

What Should I Bring In My Suitcase???

Especially if this is your first baby, you might be wondering what you should bring in your suitcase when it is time to have your baby. These days, mothers and babies are usually not in the hospital or birthing center very long after birth, but there are still some important things for you to bring.

Pack a suitcase 2 weeks before your due date and put these things in the suitcase:

- 2 or 3 nightgowns and a bathrobe (even though you might go home in a day or two, nightgowns can get messy after birth and you need clean ones)
- Slippers
- 2 bras (if you will be breast-feeding, buy nursing bras)
- A comb, a brush, a toothbrush, toothpaste, make-up, etc.

Don't bring any expensive jewelry, credit cards, or much cash with you. There might not be any safe place to keep these things.

Your baby needs to ride in a baby car seat on the way home. Your baby is not safe riding in your arms in a car. Have a family member bring a baby car seat when you go home.

Pack your baby's clothes, and let your family bring those things on the day you are going home. Put these things in the baby's suitcase:

- Diapers (and safety pins if you are using cloth diapers)
- An undershirt and an outfit for the baby to wear home
- A sweater and hat
- A light (receiving) blanket and a heavy baby blanket if it is cold outside

Flesch-Kincaid Reading Level: 4.8

Special Instructions _____

_____

_____

_____

_____

Phone number to call if you have questions: _____

Copyright © Lippincott Williams & Wilkins. Developed by MC Freda, EdD, RN, CHES, FAAN.

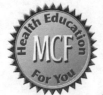

Woman's name: _____

Date: _____

Nurse's name: _____

¿¿¿Qué Es Lo Que Debo Traer En Mi Maleta???

Especialmente si es su primer bebé, se debe estar preguntando que es lo que debe traer en su maleta cuando es tiempo de dar a luz. Estos días las madres y bebés no se quedan normalmente en el hospital ó centro de parto por mucho tiempo después del parto pero todavía hay algunas cosas importantes que debe traer.

Empaque su maleta 2 semanas antes de que sea su día de dar a luz y ponga estas cosas en la maleta:

- 2 o 3 batas de dormir y una bata de baño (a pesar de que se vaya a casa en uno o dos días, batas de dormir se pueden ensuciar después del parto y necesitará algunas limpias)
- Sandalias
- 2 sostenes (si va a dar de mamar, compre sostenes de lactancia)
- Un peine, cepillo, cepillo de dientes, pasta de dientes, maquillaje, etc.

No traiga joyas, tarjetas de crédito, o demasiado dinero consigo. Pueda que no haya ningún lugar seguro donde poner estas cosas.

Su bebé necesitará viajar en una silla para bebés de carro en rumbo a casa. Su bebé no estará seguro viajando en sus brazos en el carro. Haga que un miembro de su familia traiga una silla de bebé cuando regrese a casa.

Empaque la ropa de su bebé y deje que su familia traiga esas cosas en el día que regrese a casa. Ponga estas cosas en la maleta del bebé:

- Pañales (e imperdibles si está usando pañales de algodón)
- Una camisa interior y ropa para que el bebé lo use cuando vaya a casa
- Un sweater y sombrero
- Una frazada de bebé delgada y otra más gruesa si es que hace frío afuera

Special Instructions _____

_____

_____

_____

Phone number to call if you have questions: _____

Copyright © Lippincott Williams & Wilkins. Developed by MC Freda, EdD, RN, CHES, FAAN.

Are You In Labor? How Do You Know When To Call Or Come To The Hospital or Birthing Center?

Labor is different for every woman. It's hard, therefore, to give rules that every woman should follow. There are some general rules, but if you have any question or you are concerned about anything at all, call your doctor, midwife, or nurse. They will answer your specific questions.

In general, this is when you should call or come to the hospital or birthing center:

- When your contractions are 5 minutes apart and last about 1 minute each and have been that way for about 1 hour.
- Call your doctor, nurse, or midwife if your water breaks in a big gush or you feel water trickling out of your vagina. He or she might tell you to wait at home for labor to start, but he or she needs to know that your water has broken.
- If you have bleeding like a period. This can be dangerous, so have someone call and tell your provider while you go to the hospital right away. This is different from the ``bloody show,'' which is a discharge with light spotting and mucus. Bloody show is normal.
- If you have very sharp pain in your abdomen that doesn't go away. Contractions come and go, like cramps, but pain that doesn't go away can be dangerous.
- If you can't stop vomiting, go to the hospital or birthing center.
- If you have a severe headache that won't go away, go to the hospital or birthing center.
- If the baby stops moving, or is moving very little, go to the hospital or birthing center.
- If you develop a fever, call your provider or go to the hospital.

It is always better to call and speak to your doctor, nurse, or midwife than to wait at home many hours wondering if everything is okay.

Flesch-Kincaid Reading Level: 6.3

Special Instructions _____

_____

_____

_____

_____

Phone number to call if you have questions: _____

Copyright © Lippincott Williams & Wilkins. Developed by MC Freda, EdD, RN, CHES, FAAN.

Health Education For You MCF

Woman's name: _____

Date: _____

Nurse's name: _____

¿Dolores de parto? ¿Cómo sabes cuando debes llamar o ir al hospital o centro de maternidad?

El parto es diferente para cada mujer. Por lo tanto, es difícil que hayan reglas fijas para cada mujer. Existen unas reglas generales, pero si tienes alguna pregunta, o estás preocupada por algo, llama a tu doctor, comadrona o enfermera. Ellos responderán a tus preguntas.

En general, estas son señales que te indican cuando tienes que ir al hospital ó centro de maternidad:

- Cuando tienes contracciones cada 5 minutos y duran por lo menos un minuto cada una, y has permanecido así por lo menos por una hora.
- Llama a tu doctor, enfermera o comadrona, cuando la fuente de agua se rompa o que sientas que está saliendo agua de tu vagina. Ellos te podrían decir que esperes en casa hasta que el parto comience, pero ellos necesitan saber si se rompió la fuente de agua.
- Si has sangrado como si tuvieras tu período. Esto puede ser peligroso, así que otra persona debe llamar y hablar con tu doctor mientras que tu te vas hacia el hospital. Esto es muy diferente al "moco sangriento" el cual es un flujo con rasgos de sangre y mucosidad. Esto es normal.
- Si has sentido un dolor muy agudo en tu abdomen y no se te alivia. Contracciones van y vienen, como calambres, pero dolor que no se alivia puede ser peligroso.
- Si no paras de vomitar, vé al hospital o centro de maternidad.
- Si tienes fuerte dolor de cabeza y no se te alivia, ve al hospital o centro de maternidad.
- Si el bebé para de moverse o se mueve poco, ve al hospital o centro de maternidad.
- Si tienes fiebre, llama a tu doctor o ve al hospital

Siempre es mejor llamar y hablar con tu doctor, enfermera ó comadrona que esperar en casa por muchas horas y preguntándote si todo marcha bien.

Special Instructions _____

_____

_____

_____

_____

Phone number to call if you have questions: _____

Copyright © Lippincott Williams & Wilkins. Developed by MC Freda, EdD, RN, CHES, FAAN.

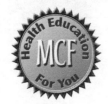

Woman's name: _____

Date: _____

Nurse's name: _____

Your Rights and Responsibilities in Labor

Some of your rights:

You have the right to have a person you choose be with you during labor to give you support.

You have the right to know the names of all the people who are caring for you.

After your doctor, nurse, or midwife explains your choices, you have the right to make your own decisions about pain relief and anesthesia.

You have the right to be told everything that the providers are doing for you and your baby.

You have the right to refuse any treatments you don't want.

You have the right to see your baby being born.

If the baby is healthy, you have the right to breast-feed as soon as you give birth if you want to.

You have the right to keep your baby with you after the birth unless the baby needs special care.

You have the right to speak to the providers who will be caring for your baby.

Some of your responsibilities:

If you have a particular philosophy about birth, you are responsible for choosing a birthing site and provider with a similar philosophy to yours (use of fetal monitoring, IVs, children visiting, anesthesia, etc.).

You are responsible for contacting your provider and finding out when to come to the hospital or birthing center.

You are responsible for learning the rules about the place you will give birth (who can come with you, eating or drinking while in labor, visiting hours, videotaping, whether the baby can be kept in your room, etc.).

During your labor, you are responsible for listening to what your doctor, midwife, or nurse suggests, and then deciding what you want.

You are responsible for asking questions when you don't understand what is being done for you or for the baby.

Flesch-Kincaid Reading Level: 8.1

Special Instructions _____

_____

_____

Phone number to call if you have questions: _____

Copyright © Lippincott Williams & Wilkins. Developed by MC Freda, EdD, RN, CHES, FAAN.

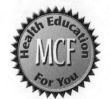

Woman's name: _____

Date: _____

Nurse's name: _____

Derechos y Responsabilidades en el Parto

Algunos de tus derechos:

Tienes el derecho de tener una persona que hayas escogido durante el parto para darte soporte.

Tienes el derecho de saber los nombres de todas las personas que estén atendiéndote.

Después que el doctor, enfermera o comadrona te hayan explicado sobre los métodos de anestesia o diferentes medicamentos para el dolor, tienes el derecho de escoger y tomar tu decisión sobre la anestesia y medicamentos para el dolor.

Tienes el derecho de que se te informe todo lo referente sobre lo que los doctores estan haciendo por tí y tu bebé.

Tienes el derecho de rechazar cualquier tratamiento que no quieras.

Tienes el derecho de ver a tu bebé nacer.

Si el bebé es saludable, tienes el derecho de amamantarlo tan pronto nazca y si así lo deseas.

Tienes el derecho de mantener el bebé contigo después del nacimiento a menos que el bebé necesite cuidados especiales.

Tienes el derecho de hablar con los doctores quienes cuidarán a tu bebé.

Algunas de tus responsabilidades:

Si tienes alguna filosofía particular sobre el nacimiento, eres responsable de escoger un lugar y doctor que comparta la misma filosofía que tu (uso del monitor fetal, intra-venosa, visitas de niños, anestesia., etc).

Eres responsable por ponerte en contacto con tu doctor y averiguar cuando tienes que ir al hospital o centro de maternidad.

Eres responsable de aprender las reglas sobre el lugar donde darás a luz (quien se puede quedar contigo, comer o tomar durante el parto, horas de visita, cámara de video, si el bebé se puede quedar en el cuarto con la madre, etc.).

Durante el parto, eres responsable de eschuchar las sugerencias de tu doctor, comadrona, o enfermera y luego tomar una decisión sobre lo que deseas.

Eres responsable de hacer preguntas cuando no entiendas lo que se está haciendo por tí y por tu bebé.

Special Instructions _____

_____

_____

_____

Phone number to call if you have questions: _____

Copyright © Lippincott Williams & Wilkins. Developed by MC Freda, EdD, RN, CHES, FAAN.

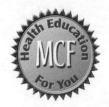

Woman's name: _____

Date: _____

Nurse's name: _____

Questions to Ask Your Provider About Labor

If you're like most women, you're worried about labor. That's normal. If this is your first baby, or if your provider, hospital, or birthing center is new to you, you really don't know what to expect. You should read the questions on this page and the next page, and decide which ones are important to you. Some of them might not interest you, and that's okay. Choose the questions you want answers for, and ask your provider to answer them for you.

Questions about recognizing labor

When should I call you if I think I'm in labor?

Should I come to the hospital or birthing center as soon as I start to feel contractions?

What do I do if my water breaks at home?

What is the mucus plug?

What is a "bloody show?"

How do I know if I'm bleeding too much?

Questions about hospital or birthing center policies for labor

Who can be with me during my labor and birth?

Is there a limit to the number of people who can be with me?

Can my other children stay for the labor and birth?

What are the rules for having children present during labor and birth?

Can I bring a doula (a special labor helper) with me when I'm admitted?

Do I have to stay in bed when I'm in labor?

Will I be hooked up to machines monitoring me in labor?

Will I have to have an IV (needle in the vein) during labor?

Can I be sitting up when I have the baby? Can I be lying on my side?

Does your hospital or birthing center use water tubs for women in labor?

Can I have a water birth if I want one?

Can I breast-feed my baby right after birth?

Can my partner participate in the birth by cutting the cord?

Can we take pictures of the birth?

Can we take videotape of the birth?

Can my baby stay with me all the time?

Flesch-Kincaid Reading Level: 4.1

Special Instructions _____

_____

_____

Phone number to call if you have questions: _____

Copyright © Lippincott Williams & Wilkins. Developed by MC Freda, EdD, RN, CHES, FAAN.

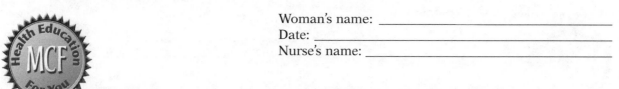

Woman's name: _____
Date: _____
Nurse's name: _____

Preguntas que le debe hacer a su Doctor acerca del Parto

Sí usted es como la mayoría de las mujeres, le preocupa el parto. Eso es normal . Si éste es su primer bebé o si su hospital o maternidad es algo nuevo para usted, en realidad no sabría que esperar. Usted debería de leer las preguntas de ésta y la siguiente página y decidir cuales son importantes para usted. No se preocupe si algunas no son de su interés, es normal. Marque las preguntas a las que desea respuestas y pídale a su doctor que se las conteste.

Preguntas de como reconocer un parto

¿Cuándo debo de avisar si pienso de que estoy por dar a luz?

¿Tan pronto sienta contracciones debería de ir al hospital?

¿Qué debo hacer si se me rompe la bolsa de agua en mi casa?

¿Qué es el tapón mucoso?

¿Qué es el sangrado vaginal?

¿Cómo puedo diferenciar entre el sangrado vaginal y el sangrado normal?

¿Cómo se si estoy sangrando demasiado?

Preguntas sobre las reglas de parto en los hospitales y maternidades

¿Quién me puede acompañar durante el parto y al dar a luz?

¿Hay un límite al número de personas que me pueden acompañar?

¿Pueden mis otros hijos acompañarme durante el parto y mientras doy a luz?

¿Cuáles son los reglamentos sobre la presencia de niños durante el parto y dar a luz?

¿Puedo traer conmigo a una ayudante cuando sea admitida?

¿Tengo que permanecer en cama durante el parto o estaré conectada a máquinas que vigilarán mi parto?

¿Tendrán que ponerme una aguja intravenosa durante el parto?

¿Me podré sentar cuando tenga a mi bebé? Me puedo acostar de lado?

¿Permiten mi hospital o maternidad de que las mujeres usen bañeras de agua durante el parto?

¿Puedo tener un nacimiento de agua si así lo deseo?

¿Puedo amamantar a mi bebé apenas nazca?

¿Puede mi acompañante participar en el parto cortando el cordón umbilical?

¿Podemos tomar fotos del nacimiento?

¿Podemos grabar en cinta el nacimiento?

¿Puede mi bebé permanecer conmigo todo el tiempo?

Special Instructions _____

_____

Phone number to call if you have questions: _____

Copyright © Lippincott Williams & Wilkins. Developed by MC Freda, EdD, RN, CHES, FAAN.

Woman's name: _____

Date: _____

Nurse's name: _____

More Questions to Ask Your Provider About Labor

If you're like most women, you're worried about labor. That's normal. If this is your first baby, or if your provider, hospital, or birthing center is new to you, you really don't know what to expect. You should read the questions on this page and the previous page and decide which ones are important to you. Some of them might not interest you, and that's okay. Choose the questions you want answers for, and ask your provider to answer them for you.

Questions about pain and pain relief in labor

Will you give me medicines to stop the pain of labor if I ask for them?

What kind of medicines do you use?

What are my options for pain relief in labor?

If I take pain medicines for labor, can I still be awake for the birth?

What if I want to go through labor with no pain medicine at all?

If I choose hypnosis for labor, do you support that?

Do you think epidural anesthesia is a good choice for pain relief in labor?

When do you usually give the epidural?

Are there special doctors or nurses at your hospital 24 hours a day who give epidural anesthesia?

Other important questions

What is your cesarean birth rate?

Do you believe in VBAC (vaginal birth after cesarean)?

What would cause you to decide an emergency cesarean birth is necessary?

What happens if my baby is breech?

How do you feel about breast-feeding?

Will you support me breast-feeding my baby immediately after birth?

If I want to go home within 24 hours after I give birth, is that possible?

Flesch-Kincaid Reading Level: 5.6

Special Instructions _____

_____

_____

_____

_____

Phone number to call if you have questions: _____

Copyright © Lippincott Williams & Wilkins. Developed by MC Freda, EdD, RN, CHES, FAAN.

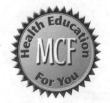

Woman's name: _____

Date: _____

Nurse's name: _____

Más Preguntas acerca del Parto que Usted le debe hacer a su Doctor

Si usted es como la mayoría de las mujeres, le preocupa el parto. Eso es normal. Si éste es su primer bebé o si su hospital o maternidad es algo nuevo para usted, en realidad no sabría que esperar. Usted debería de leer las preguntas de ésta y la siguiente página y decidir cuales son importantes para usted. No se preocupe si algunas no son de su interés, es normal. Marque las preguntas a las que desea respuestas y pídale a su doctor que se las conteste.

Preguntas acerca del dolor y su alivio durante el parto

¿Si se lo pido usted me dará medicinas para el dolor de parto?

¿Qué clase de medicamentos usa usted?

¿Durante el parto qué clase de opciones tengo para aliviar el dolor?

¿Si durante el parto tomo medicamentos para el dolor, todavía puedo estar despierta para dar a luz?

¿Qué sucede si yo deseo tener el parto sin usar ningún medicamento para el dolor?

¿Si yo deseo que me hipnotizen para el parto, ustedes me apoyarían con esto?

¿Piensa usted de que la anestesia Epidural es una buena elección para aliviar el dolor durante el parto?

¿Generalmente cuándo usted aplica la anestesia de Epidural?

¿En su hospital, hay enfermeras o doctores especiales que administren la anestesia Epidural las 24 horas del día?

Otras preguntas importantes

¿ Cuál es su promedio de nacimientos por cesárea?

¿Usted cree en el nacimiento vaginal después de una cesárea?

¿Si fuese necesario,qué la llevaría a decidirse por un parto por cesárea?

¿Qué pasa si mi bebé está de nalgas?

¿Me inducirían el parto si se lo pidiese?

¿Me apoyarían a que amamante a mi bebé inmediatamente después de que nazca?

¿ Es posible de que me vaya a mi casa dentro de las 24 horas después de haber dado a luz?

Special Instructions _____

_____

_____

_____

Phone number to call if you have questions: _____

Copyright © Lippincott Williams & Wilkins. Developed by MC Freda, EdD, RN, CHES, FAAN.

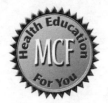

Woman's name: _____

Date: _____

Nurse's name: _____

Pain Relief for the Birth of Your Baby

Labor and the birth of your baby occur by contractions (tightening) of your womb and by the stretching of the birth canal. Most women find the contractions and stretching uncomfortable. You should discuss this with your doctor, nurse, or midwife before you go into labor so everyone knows what you want to happen.

Natural childbirth

Some women want to deliver their babies with very little or no medicine for pain relief. There are special classes you can attend during pregnancy, when instructions and exercises to aid childbirth are given. Your provider can tell you exactly when these classes are available.

Medications

Medicines can be given into your vein as one method of pain relief. These medicines should be given only by a doctor, midwife, or nurse, because too much of these medicines could affect your baby. Ask your doctor, nurse, or midwife about this.

Regional anesthesia

Another type of pain relief uses "local" anesthesia drugs (like "Novocaine") in the vagina or in the back. With this, you will be awake during the birth of your baby, but you should have little or no pain. The following are the various ways in which regional anesthesia is given:

Pudendal Block—this is given just as the baby is about to be born. The medicine is injected through the vagina by the doctor or midwife. It relieves the pain of delivery, but not labor.

Epidural Block—this medicine is given through a needle placed between two of the lowest backbones. The needle is <u>not</u> inserted deeply and does <u>not</u> enter the spine. After the skin is numb, a tiny tube (called a catheter) is put through the needle, the needle is removed, and the tube is left in place. This gives you pain relief for the labor and the birth. However, your full cooperation is necessary. You will be asked to lie on your side with your back bent or to sit up so the medicine can be injected into your lower back. Medicine is given through the tube. The tube (catheter) is removed after the birth.

Spinal Block—this medicine is injected into the fluid surrounding the lower spine. You will need to keep very still during this. Spinal block is sometimes used for cesarean sections.

General anesthesia

This pain relief, given by gas, is only used sometimes, usually in emergency situations. First you would be given oxygen through a mask placed over your face and told to breathe normally. Then you would be given other gases to help you relax and ease your pain during delivery. Sometimes you must be put completely to sleep for your delivery.

All these methods of pain relief may not be available everywhere, so be sure to ask your doctor, nurse or midwife what is available where you will give birth.

Flesch-Kincaid Reading Level: 7.8

Special Instructions _____

_____

Phone number to call if you have questions: _____

Copyright © Lippincott Williams & Wilkins. Developed by MC Freda, EdD, RN, CHES, FAAN.

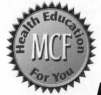

Alivio Del Dolor Para El Nacimiento De Su Bebé

El parto y el nacimiento de su bebé occurre con contracciones de su útero y el estiro de su canal de nacimiento. La mayoría de las mujeres encuentran las contracciones y el estiro incomódos. Debe discutir esto con su doctor, enfermera o partera antes de que comience el parto para que todos sepan lo que usted quiere que ocurra.

Parto natural

Algunas mujeres quieren dar a luz con muy poco o sin medicina para aliviar el dolor. Hay clases especiales que puede asistir durante su embarazo, donde se dan instrucciones y ejercicios para ayudar con el parto. Su proveedor de salud le prodrá decir exactamente cuando estas clases son disponibles.

Medicamentos

Medicamentos se pueden dar a través de sus venas como un método para aliviar el dolor. Estos medicamentos solo se deben dar por un doctor, partera o enfermera, porque mucha cantidad de estas medicinas pueden afectar su bebé. Pregúntele a su doctor, enfermera o partera sobre esto.

Anestesia regional

Otro tipo de alivio del dolor utiliza drogas de anestesia "local" (como la "novocaina") en la vagina o en la espalda. Con esto, va a estar despierta durante el parto de su bebé pero tendrá muy poco o ningún dolor. Las siguientos son las varias maneras en que la anestesia local se da:

Bloque Pudendal—esto se da justo antes que el bebé nazca. La medicina se inyecta a través de la vagina por un doctor o partera. Alivie el dolor del parto, pero no el parto.

Bloque Epidural—esta medicina se da a través de una aguja puesta entre dos de los huesos de la espalda. La aguja <u>no</u> es insertada profundamente, y <u>no</u> entra en la espina dorsal. Después que la piel esté adormecida, un pequeño tubo (llamado catéter) es puesto a través de la aguja, la aguja es removida y el tubo permanece en su lugar. Esto le dará alivio para el dolor del parto y el nacimiento. Sin embargo, su completa cooperación es necesaria. Se le pedirá que se acueste de lado con su espalda doblada, o que se siente para que la medicina pueda ser inyectada en la parte baja de su espalda. La medicina es dada a través del tubo. El tubo (cáteter) es removido después del parto.

Bloque Espinal—la medicina es inyectada en el líquido que se se encuentra alrededor de la parte baja de su espina dorsal. Necesitará que se mantenga bien quieta durante esto. El bloque espinal es a veces usado para cesarias.

Anestesia general

Este alivio del dolor es dado a través de gas, es solamente usado algunas veces, normalmente durante situaciones de emergencia. Primero, se la daría oxígeno a través de una máscara puesta sobre su cara y se le pedirá que respire normalmente. Después se le darán otros gases que le ayudarán a mejorar su dolor durante el parto.

Todos estos métodos de alivio del dolor no son disponibles en todos lados, por eso pregunte a su doctor, enfermera o partera lo que es disponible en el hospital donde va a dar a luz.

Special Instructions _____

_____

Phone number to call if you have questions: _____

Copyright © Lippincott Williams & Wilkins. Developed by MC Freda, EdD, RN, CHES, FAAN.

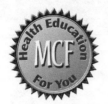
Episiotomy

What is an episiotomy?

An episiotomy (ee-peas-ee-ott-o-me) is a cut just below your vagina done by a doctor or midwife during the birth of a baby. The skin between the bottom of your vagina and your rectum is cut. This area is called your "perineum." The cut is made because the doctor or midwife feels that your baby's head might need extra room to get out during the birthing process.

Why is episiotomy done?

Until the past few years, many doctors thought that doing an episiotomy was the safest way to help a baby be born. They thought that cutting the perineum would prevent the skin from tearing.

Are episiotomies still done?

They are done much less than they used to be done. Most doctors and midwives now feel that if your labor is normal, the skin of the perineum automatically stretches enough to allow the head to be delivered without any skin tearing. Most providers today only do an episiotomy when there seems to be a specific problem such as a really large baby.

Does it hurt?

If you have an episiotomy, the doctor or midwife will numb the skin with a shot before they cut. It should not hurt. They will then sew up the episiotomy after the birth is over, and the stitches will heal in about a month. The stitches do not have to be taken out. You might feel sore for a week or two. You can use ice packs to help relieve the pain. Your doctor or midwife might tell you to take Tylenol or some other mild pain reliever. If you are breast-feeding, be sure to ask your doctor or midwife if taking pain medicine is a good idea. You have to be sure to keep that area clean so it heals well.

You should ask your doctor or midwife what they think about episiotomy and what you can expect during the birth of your baby.

Flesch-Kincaid Reading Level: 6.9

Special Instructions _____

_____

_____

Phone number to call if you have questions: _____

Copyright © Lippincott Williams & Wilkins. Developed by MC Freda, EdD, RN, CHES, FAAN.

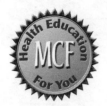

Woman's name: _____

Date: _____

Nurse's name: _____

Episitomía

¿Qué es una episitomía?

Una episitomía es un corte por debajo de la vagina hecho por un doctor o comadrona durante el nacimiento de un bebé. La piel dentro de la parte inferior de la vagina y el recto es cortada. Esta área es llamada "perineo". El corte es hecho porque el doctor piensa que la cabeza del bebé necesitará espacio extra para salir durante el proceso del nacimiento.

¿Por qué es hecha una episitomía?

Hasta hace unos años atrás, muchos doctores pensaban que el hacer una episitomía era la forma más segura de ayudar a un bebé para nacer. Ellos pensaban que al cortar el "perineo" ayudaría a que la piel no se rasgara.

¿Todavía se hace el procedimiento de la episitomía?

Estas son hechas en menor escala comparado a la cantidad que se hacían anteriormente. Actualmente muchos doctores y comadronas piensan que si el proceso del parto es normal, la piel del perineo automaticamente se extiende lo suficiente para que la cabeza del bebé salga sin que la piel se rasgue. Hoy en día, muchos proveedores sólo hacen la episitomía cuando hay un problema específico como el de un bebé muy grande.

¿Duele el procedimiento?

Si le van a hacer una episitomía, el doctor o una comadrona le adormecerá la piel con una inyección antes de hacer la incisión. No tendrá dolor. Luego le tomaran unos puntos después del nacimiento del bebé. Los puntos se curaran en un mes. Los puntos no necesitan que se quiten. Usted se sentirá un poco adolorida por una semana o dos. Puede usar paquetes de hielo para aliviar el dolor. Si estás amamantando es un buena idea que le preguntes al doctor si puedes tomar alguna medicina para aliviar el dolor. Tiene que asegurarse de mantener el área limpia y seca para que se cure totalmente.

Pregúntele a su doctor o comadroma sobre lo que piensa sobre la episitomía, y que puede usted esperar durante el nancimiento de su bebé.

Special Instructions _____

_____

Phone number to call if you have questions: _____

Copyright © Lippincott Williams & Wilkins. Developed by MC Freda, EdD, RN, CHES, FAAN.

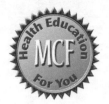

Woman's name: _____

Date: _____

Nurse's name: _____

Water Tubs in Labor

Water has been used for hundreds of years to treat pain. Recently many institutions (hospitals and birthing centers) have begun to use water tubs for women in labor to decrease the pain of labor contractions. Several studies have shown that women who labor in a water tub use less medicine for pain and feel very satisfied with their labor experience. Using a water tub for labor is different from giving birth when in the water.

Are you interested in using a water tub during labor?

If you are, you need to find out if the hospital or birthing center you have chosen for your birthing experience offers this treatment. You should ask your doctor, midwife, or nurse about this. Usually only women who are healthy and who have normal, uncomplicated pregnancies at term will labor in a water tub. You will probably have to have a support person with you at all times (that is, a husband, significant other, mother, sister, friend).

What will happen at the hospital or birthing center?

- If your institution offers water tubs, you can expect that all the nurses on the staff will understand their safe use.
- The tubs are cleaned thoroughly after each woman uses them.
- The water temperature should be between 96F to 105F.
- You will probably use the tub only after your cervix has reached about 5 cm dilation.
- The nurses will probably listen to the baby's heartbeat and take your blood pressure every 30 minutes. You might be assisted out of the tub for these assessments.
- If your water breaks, your provider will decide if you may still use the water tub.
- In many institutions, you do not actually give birth in the water, but move to a labor bed for the birth.

Be sure that your support person stays with you all the time you're in the water tub. If at any time you feel too hot, or like you might faint, your support person should call for help by using the intercom, not by leaving you and going to get a nurse.

Flesch-Kincaid Reading Level: 6.9

Special Instructions _____

_____

_____

_____

Phone number to call if you have questions: _____

Copyright © Lippincott Williams & Wilkins. Developed by MC Freda, EdD, RN, CHES, FAAN.

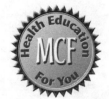

Woman's name: _____

Date: _____

Nurse's name: _____

El Uso de la Bañera en los Partos

Por cientos de años las bañeras de agua han sido usadas para tratar el dolor. Recientemente muchas instituciones (hospitales y maternidades) han empezado a usar las bañeras en los partos de las mujeres para disminuir el dolor de las contracciones del parto. Varios estudios han demostrado de que las mujeres que dan a luz usando las bañeras, usan menos medicinas para el dolor y se sienten muy conformes con su experiencia de sus partos. El uso de la bañera para partos es diferente a dar el parto mientras esté en el agua. En muchas de las instituciones donde se utiliza la bañera para el parto se traslada a la mujer a una cama de parto para que dé a luz.

¿Esta usted interesada en usar una bañera durante su parto?

Si lo está, usted necesita averiguar si el hospital o maternidad que escogió para dar a luz le ofrece este tipo de tratamiento. Debería de consultar con su doctor, comadrona o enfermera. Generalmente sólo aquellas mujeres que esten saludable, y que tienen embarazos normales y sin complicaciones, podran usar las bañera de agua para el parto. Es muy posible de que usted tenga la necesidad de tener una persona que la apoye todo el tiempo (tal como su esposo, mamá, hermana o amistad).

¿Qué pasará en el hospital o maternidad?

- Si su institución ofrece bañeras de agua, puede contar con que el personal de enfermeras las sepan manejar de una manera segura.
- Las bañeras son completamente aseadas después de cada uso.
- Probablemente usted usará la bañera después de que su útero haya dilatado 5 centímetros.
- Probablemente su enfermera escuchará los latidos del corazón de su bebé y le tomará la presión cada 30 minutos. Le ayudaran a salir de la bañera para hacerles estas pruebas.
- Si se le rompe la bolsa de agua, su doctor decidirá si usted todavía necesita usar la bañera.
- En realidad, en muchas de las instituciones, usted no dá a luz dentro del agua sino que la llevan a una cama de parto para que dé a luz.

Asegúrese de que su persona de apoyo se quede con usted todo el tiempo que permanezca en la bañera Si en algún momento se siente muy caliente o se siente desmayar su persona de apoyo deberá de pedir ayuda usando el intercomunicador o apretando el botón encendido y no debe de dejarla sola para ir a buscar a la enfermera.

Special Instructions _____

_____

Phone number to call if you have questions: _____

Copyright © Lippincott Williams & Wilkins. Developed by MC Freda, EdD, RN, CHES, FAAN.

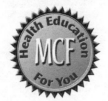

Woman's name: _____

Date: _____

Nurse's name: _____

Photographing and Videotaping Your Birth

Many people want to videotape their labor and birth experience. Keeping that memory forever is important to them. Other people just want to take regular pictures. What many people do not know, however, is that not all institutions allow videotaping or picture taking.

Does your institution allow videotaping and picture taking?

When you are choosing your provider, you should know that most providers only do deliveries at one hospital or birthing center. That means you have no choice about the hospital or birthing center where you will have your baby. You must go where your provider goes. If that place has rules you don't like, you have a problem!

Some institutions allow picture taking and videotaping, and others do not. Some allow you to videotape anything you like, but many institutions have rules about when videotaping can be done and who can be in the pictures.

What should you do if you want to videotape?

If you have been planning on videotaping your labor and birth, it could be very upsetting for you to arrive at the labor area and find out you are not allowed you to do so! So, ask your doctor or midwife early in your pregnancy what the rules are where you will be giving birth. If you do not agree with the rules, you'll have to decide whether you want to change providers and institutions to find a place that allows you to videotape.

It is always better to be prepared and understand what is expected of you. Make a list of what is important to you during labor, and go over it with your provider.

Flesch-Kincaid Reading Level: 8.0

Special Instructions _____

_____

_____

_____

_____

_____

Phone number to call if you have questions: _____

Copyright © Lippincott Williams & Wilkins. Developed by MC Freda, EdD, RN, CHES, FAAN.

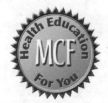

Woman's name: _____

Date: _____

Nurse's name: _____

Filmando y Fotografiando su Nacimiento

Muchas personas desean grabar su experiencia durante su parto y nacimiento.Mantenerlo por siempre en su recuerdo es una cosa muy importante para ellos. Otras personas sólo prefieren tomar fotos. Lo que muchas personas no saben es de que no todas las instituciones permiten que se tomen fotos o que se hagan grabaciones en video.

¿Le permite su hospital tomar fotos o grabación en video?

Cuando esté seleccionando a su doctor , debería de saber de que la mayoría solamente atienden los partos en hospitales o centros de nacimiento. Esto quiere decir de que usted no podrá escoger el hospital o centro de maternidad donde su hijo(a) nacerá. Usted debe de ir donde su doctor se lo indique. Si ése lugar tiene reglas que no son de su agrado, tendrá un problema.

Algunos hospitales le permiten de que grabe y tome fotos, en cambio otros nó. Algunos le permiten de que grabe lo que usted desee, otros le diran cuando usted puede grabar y quienes pueden estar en la foto.

¿Qué deberá hacer si usted desea grabar en video?

Debe de ser bien frustrante el llegar al área de parto y que no le permitan grabarlo después de haberlo así planeado. De tal manera pregúntele a su doctor o comadrona, durante el inicio de su embarazo, sobre las reglas que rigen en el lugar donde usted va a dar a luz. Si usted no está de acuerdo con las reglas, tendrá que decidir si cambiar o nó de doctor o hospital y buscar un lugar que le permitan grabaciones en video.

Es mejor estar siempre preparado y comprender que se espera de usted. Prepare una lista indicando que es lo más importante para usted y revísela con su doctor.

Special Instructions _____

_____

_____

_____

_____

_____

Phone number to call if you have questions: _____

Copyright © Lippincott Williams & Wilkins. Developed by MC Freda, EdD, RN, CHES, FAAN.

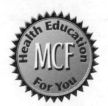

Woman's name: _____

Date: _____

Nurse's name: _____

Cesarean Birth

Cesarean birth is sometimes called "Cesarean Section." In a cesarean birth, the baby is removed from the womb during an operation through the abdomen and into the uterus. Cesarean operations are usually done when there is an emergency and either the baby must be delivered quickly to save its life or the mother cannot give birth vaginally.

In the United States about 25% of babies are born this way. The rates are different at each hospital and in different parts of the country. You should ask your doctor, nurse, or midwife about the cesarean birth rates at the hospital where you will have your baby.

Women with the following problems may be at higher risk of having a cesarean birth:

Diabetes
High blood pressure
Certain vaginal infections
Breech position of the baby
Fetal distress (meaning the baby needs to be delivered right away)
Placenta previa (when the afterbirth is between the baby and the cervix)
A labor that does not progress normally

Cesarean birth is an operation, and all operations can be dangerous, so they should only be done when absolutely necessary. It is important that you talk to your doctor, nurse, or midwife about this when you are still pregnant. Tell him or her that you would like to be involved in the decision should cesarean become necessary. If you are prepared for the possibility of cesarean birth and know what to expect, cesarean birth does not have to be so scary.

It used to be that if you had a cesarean birth once, then all of your births had to be by Cesarean. That is not necessarily true today. Now there is **"VBAC"** (pronounced "V-back"). This means "vaginal birth after cesarean." A great deal of research has been done on VBAC, and it has been found to be a safe way to have a baby for most women. Find out if your doctor or midwife thinks VBAC would be a good choice for you this time. If you choose VBAC, be sure to attend childbirth education classes so you and your partner are prepared for labor.

Flesch-Kincaid Reading Level: 7.1

Special Instructions _____

_____

_____

Phone number to call if you have questions: _____

Copyright © Lippincott Williams & Wilkins. Developed by MC Freda, EdD, RN, CHES, FAAN.

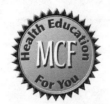

Woman's name: _____

Date: _____

Nurse's name: _____

Parto Por Cesárea

En un parto por cesárea, el bebé es removido del vientre de la madre durante una operación a través del abdomen y dentro del útero. Las operaciones por cesárea son generalmente hechas en caso de emergencia o cuando el bebé debe ser removido rápidamente para salvar su vida o cuando la madre no puede dar a luz vaginalmente.

En los Estados Unidos cerca del 25% de los bebés nacen de esta forma. Las estadísticas son diferentes en cada hospital y en diferente partes del país. Deberías preguntarle a tu doctor, enfermera o comadrona sobre los índices de parto por cesárea en el hospital donde vas a dar a luz.

Mujeres con alto riesgo de tener un parto por Cesárea:

Diábetes

Presión arterial alta

Ciertas infecciones vaginales

Bebé en mala posición (sentado)

Estrés fetal (el bebé necesita nacer de immediato)

Placenta previa (cuando la placenta se encuentra entre el bebé y el cervix)

Un parto que no progresa normalmente.

Parto por cesárea es una operación, y como todas las operaciones, puede ser peligrosas, así que deben ser hechas cuando sea absolutamente necesaria. Es importante que usted hable con su doctor, enfermera o comadrona sobre esto mientras este embarazada. Dígale que le gustaría participar en la decisión de tener o no una cesárea. Si estas preparada para la posibilidad de un parto por cesárea y entiendes lo que se puede esperar del procedimiento, no tendrás mayor problema y no habría la necesidad de tener miedo.

Se solía pensar que cuando una mujer tenía un parto por cesárea la primera vez, entonces todos los partos siguientes tenían que ser por cesárea también. Hoy en día ésto no es necesariamente verdad. Ahora existe algo que se llama "Parto Vaginal después de la Cesárea" Una gran cantidad de estudios se han hechos sobre ésto y demuenstran que es seguro para las mayorías de las mujeres.

Pregúntale a tu doctor o comadrona si piensa que el parto vaginal después de la cesárea es una opción para tí. Si escoges éste procedimiento, asegúrate de atender clases de educación sobre el nacimiento, de ésta forma tú y tu pareja estarán preparados para cuando llegue la hora del parto.

Special Instructions _____

_____

_____

Phone number to call if you have questions: _____

Copyright © Lippincott Williams & Wilkins. Developed by MC Freda, EdD, RN, CHES, FAAN.

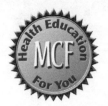

Becoming a Mother

What will you feel when you see your baby?

Some women develop strong maternal feelings when they are pregnant, but some women don't, and that's okay. Some women fall in love with their babies immediately when they see them right after birth, but some don't. For some women, falling in love with their baby takes time. It happens after they have had time to get to know and take care of the baby. The important thing for you to remember is that there isn't one particular way for all women to "become a mother." Becoming a mother happens at all different points during pregnancy and the first few weeks of life. Whenever it happens for you, that's okay. Don't feel upset if you only feel afraid, or confused after your baby is born. You might just need a little more time to get to know your baby.

Some of the things you might feel

Although women don't talk about this a lot, you might feel some of these things when you see your new baby:

- Afraid you won't be a good mother
- Afraid you won't be able to take care of the baby
- Worried about the things you are giving up to become a mother
- Think the baby looks strange (pointed head, swollen eyes, etc.)
- Can't imagine that the baby is really yours
- Disappointed in the sex of the baby

What should you do about your feelings?

- If you feel any of those things, don't be upset. You can let yourself feel it, and then it will be over.
- Talk to your nurse or midwife about your fears. He or she can help you understand that most women are afraid, even if they don't admit it!
- Learn all you can about taking care of your baby.
- Ask your family to help you at home with the housework, so you can just concentrate on taking care of your baby.

Soon you will know your baby, and taking care of your child every day will show you that you can do it. You will also begin to fall in love with your baby as the days go on. Soon you'll be bragging that you have the most beautiful and smartest baby in the world. That's all part of becoming a mother!

Flesch-Kincaid Reading Level: 4.9

Special Instructions _____

Phone number to call if you have questions: _____

Copyright © Lippincott Williams & Wilkins. Developed by MC Freda, EdD, RN, CHES, FAAN.

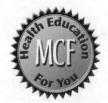

Woman's name: _____

Date: _____

Nurse's name: _____

Convertirse en Madre

¿Qué sentirá al ver a su bebé?

Algunas mujeres desarrollan un fuerte instinto maternal al salir embarazadas, otras mujeres no son así, pero ésto es normal. Algunas mujeres se enamoran de sus bebés tan pronto los ven al nacer, sin embargo, otras nó. Para algunas mujeres encariñarse con sus bebés, les toma tiempo. Esto sucede después que han tenido tiempo de conocer y haber cuidado a su bebé. Lo más importante es recordar que no hay una forma particular de convertirse en mamá. Pueda ser que el ser mamá se realice en diferente etapas del embarazo y las primeras semanas de vida del bebé. Cuando quiera que te suceda, está bien. No se desespere si siente miedo, o confundida después que el bebé haya nacido. Probablemente necesite un poquito más de tiempo para llegar a conocer a su bebé.

Algunas cosas que podías sentir

Aunque muchas mujeres no hablan mucho sobre ésto, usted podría experimentar algunas de éstas cosas cuando vea a su nuevo bebé:

- Miedo de que no sea una buena mama
- Miedo de que no cuide bien a sus bebé
- Preocupada por las cosas que tendrá que dejar de hacer para convertirte en madre.
- Piensa que el bebé luce extraño (cabeza puntiaguda, ojos hinchados, etc)
- No puede imaginarse que éste bebé es realmente suyo
- Desilusionada con el sexo del bebé.

¿Qué debo hacer sobre mis sentimientos?

- Si sientes algunas de éstas cosas, no te molestes. Déjate llevar por tus emociones y luego todo pasará.
- Comunícale a tu enfermera o comadrona sobre tus temores. Ellas te explicarán que muchas mujeres se sienten con miedo,aunque ellas no lo admitan!
- Aprende todo lo que puedas sobre el cuidado de tu bebé.
- Pídale a tu familia que te ayuden con los quehaceres del hogar, de ésta forma te concentrarás más en el cuidado del bebé.

Pronto conocerás a tu bebé, y cuidando a su bebé todos los días te demostrará que sí lo puedes hacer. También comienza a querer a tu bebé a medida que transcurren los días. Pronto te jactarás de tener el bebé más hermoso e inteligente en el mundo. ¡Todo esto es parte de convertirse en mamá!

Special Instructions _____

Phone number to call if you have questions: _____

Copyright © Lippincott Williams & Wilkins. Developed by MC Freda, EdD, RN, CHES, FAAN.

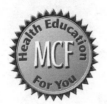

MCF
Health Education
For You

Woman's name: _____

Date: _____

Nurse's name: _____

What If Your Due Date Was Last Week?

Is it okay to go past your due date?

Very few babies are born on their due date. It is normal to give birth between 2 weeks before your due date until 2 weeks after your due date. That's between 38 weeks and 42 weeks of pregnancy. If you have gone past your due date, don't worry. Most women who do will give birth by 41 weeks. The rest will give birth by 42 weeks. Only 2% of women don't go into labor by 42 weeks.

What can go wrong if you go past 42 weeks?

It really isn't healthy for the baby to stay in your uterus after 42 weeks. The placenta (also called the "afterbirth") stops doing its job of nourishing the baby after 42 weeks. The baby can then become sick and lose weight. If you haven't gone into labor by 42 weeks, then your doctor or midwife will want to induce your labor so the baby can be born.

Should I have an induced labor if I go past my due date?

It is not necessary to induce labor until 42 weeks. The large majority of women will give birth before that. When labor is induced, strong drugs must be used that can have many side effects. It is always better to wait until 42 weeks for labor to start naturally than to induce your labor just because your due date has arrived. If you have not gone into labor by 42 weeks, then induced labor is the right choice.

Flesch-Kincaid Reading Level: 4.6

Special Instructions _____

_____

_____

_____

_____

_____

Phone number to call if you have questions: _____

Copyright © Lippincott Williams & Wilkins. Developed by MC Freda, EdD, RN, CHES, FAAN.

Woman's name: _____
Date: _____
Nurse's name: _____

¿Qué pasa si su fecha de dar a luz se venció la semana pasada?

¿Está bien si se ha pasado su fecha de dar a luz?

Muy pocos bebés nacen en la fecha asignada. Es normal dar a luz dos semanas antes o dos semanas después de su fecha asignada. Eso es entre el final de la 37ma y el final de la 42ma semanas de embarazo. No se alarme si usted se ha pasado su fecha asignada. La mayoría de las mujeres darán a luz a las cuarenta y una semanas. El resto dará a luz a las cuarenta y dos semanas. Solamente el 2% de las mujeres no dan a luz a las cuarenta y dos semanas.

¿Qué puede suceder si se pasa las cuarenta y dos semanas?

En realidad no es saludable para su bebé el quedarse dentro de su útero después de las cuarenta y dos semanas. La placenta cesa su trabajo de alimentar el bebé después de las cuarenta y dos semanas. Luego el bebé se puede enfermar y perder peso. Si usted no empieza a tener dolores de parto dentro de las cuarenta y dos semanas, entonces su doctor o comadrona querrán inducirle el parto paraque nazca su bebé .

¿Si me paso la fecha de dar a luz me deben de inducir el parto?

No es necesario de que le induzcan el parto hasta las cuarenta y dos semanas. La mayor parte de las mujeres darán a luz antes de éso. Cuando se induce el parto se usan fuertes drogas y ésto puede tener efectos secundarios. Siempre es mejor esperar hasta las cuarenta y dos semanas para que el parto empiece naturalmente; a que inducirlo sólo porque no ha llegado su fecha del parto. Si usted no ha tenido dolores de parto al cabo de las cuarenta y dos semanas entonces el parto por inducción sería lo más favorable.

Special Instructions _____

_____

_____

_____

_____

_____

Phone number to call if you have questions: _____

Copyright © Lippincott Williams & Wilkins. Developed by MC Freda, EdD, RN, CHES, FAAN.

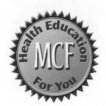

Woman's name: _____

Date: _____

Nurse's name: _____

Induction of Labor

What is induction of labor?

Induction of labor means that the doctor or midwife starts your labor with medicines or by breaking your bag of waters instead of waiting for your labor to start naturally.

Why is labor induced?

- Sometimes the baby becomes sick during pregnancy and must be born to be treated.
- Sometimes the mother becomes sick during pregnancy, and the only way she can get better is to deliver the baby.
- Sometimes the woman does not go into labor by 42 weeks of pregnancy. After 42 weeks the afterbirth stops working as well to nourish the baby. The baby can become sick and lose weight.
- Sometimes the woman has a history of very short labors, and the provider is worried that she won't make it to the hospital on time for the birth.

How is labor induced?

There are several ways. Sometimes the doctor or midwife will break your bag of waters and labor will start several hours later. Sometimes the doctor or midwife will put medicine into your vagina to "ripen" your cervix and get your uterus ready for labor. Sometimes the doctor will give you medicine through a needle into a vein in your arm to start your labor.

Is induction of labor a good thing?

If your health or the health of the baby is in question, and inducing your labor is the best thing, then induction is good. You need to discuss this with your doctor or midwife to be sure you understand exactly what will be done.

There is a lot of controversy about induction of labor done for convenience of either the mother or the provider. Many people feel that induction should only be done when there is a strong medical reason for it. That is because a natural labor that begins on its own is always the best kind of labor. It's hard to wait for labor to begin, but it is healthier for everyone. There is always the chance of something going wrong when medicines are given. These are strong medicines that can cause your uterus to rupture if you are not watched very closely during the induction. Therefore, unless your health or the baby's health is at stake, it's better to wait for your labor to begin on its own.

Flesch-Kincaid Reading Level: 7.5

Special Instructions _____

Phone number to call if you have questions: _____

Copyright © Lippincott Williams & Wilkins. Developed by MC Freda, EdD, RN, CHES, FAAN.

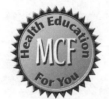

Woman's name: _____

Date: _____

Nurse's name: _____

Inducción del Parto

¿Qué es una inducción del parto?

Una inducción del parto significa de que el doctor o comadrona empieza el parto mediante el uso de medicinas, o rompiendo la bolsa de agua en vez de esperar que el parto empieze naturalmente.

¿Por qué se induce un parto?

- Algunas veces el bebé se enferma durante el embarazo y debe de nacer para ser curado.
- Algunas veces la madre se enferma durante el embarazo, y la única manera que se pueda mejorar es teniendo al bebé.
- Algunas veces la mujer no tiene dolores de parto a las cuarenta y dos semanas de embarazo. Después de las cuarenta y dos semanas la placenta no funciona muy bien al nutrir al bebé. El bebé se puede enfermar y perder peso.
- Algunas veces la mujer puede tener dolores de parto muy cortos de tal manera de que su doctor se preocupe de que ella no pueda llegar a tiempo al hospital para dar a luz.

¿Cómo se induce el parto?

Hay varias maneras. Algunas veces su doctor o comadrona le romperán su bolsa de agua y el parto comenzará varias hora después. Algunas veces el doctor, enfermera o comadrona le pondran una inyección en su vagina para que su cervix "madure" y tenga su útero listo para el parto. Algunas veces su doctor le pondrá una inyección con medicinas en las venas de su brazo para así iniciar el parto.

¿Es bueno la inducción del parto?

Si su salud o la del bebé estan en duda y la inducción del parto es la mejor alternativa; entonces la inducción es buena. Usted debe de hablar sobre ésto con su doctor o comadrona para asegurarse de que comprende exactamente lo que se vá hacer.

Existe mucha controversia sobre la inducción del parto hecha por conveniencia por parte de la madre o del doctor. Muchas personas piensan que la inducción solamente se debe hacer por motivos médicos. Esto es porque un parto natural el cual se inicia por si mismo es siempre la major manera de dar a luz. Es difícil esperar el inicio del parto sin embargo es lo más saludable para todos. Siempre existe la posibilidad de que halgo salga mal cuando se toman medicamentos. Estas son medicinas fuertes y que pueden causar la ruptura de su útero si no se le observa bien de cerca durante la inducción. Por consiguiente, a menos de que su salud corra peligro, lo mejor es esperar a que el parto empieze por sí mismo.

Special Instructions _____

Phone number to call if you have questions: _____

Copyright © Lippincott Williams & Wilkins. Developed by MC Freda, EdD, RN, CHES, FAAN.

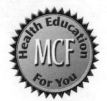

Woman's name: _____
Date: _____
Nurse's name: _____

Circumcision Is Your Decision

Circumcision is a surgery on male infants, in which the skin covering the head of the penis (called the "foreskin") is removed. The American Academy of Pediatrics (1999) has stated that it cannot recommend routine circumcision because there is no medical necessity for it. Many people, however, believe that circumcision is the right thing to do. There are no clear answers. You will be asked to decide if you wish your newborn son to have a circumcision. This information sheet will provide you with some of the things you should consider. Be sure to discuss this with your doctor, midwife, nurse, and pediatrician as well. Be sure to find out also if your insurance covers circumcision.

Why People Do It

Religious or cultural tradition

Family tradition, such as the child's father or male siblings being circumcised

Personal beliefs, for example, a belief that the circumcised penis is easier to keep clean, or that circumcised males have better sexual performance

If circumcision is done later in life it requires being admitted to the hospital

Some researchers suggest that cancer of the penis, although a rare disease, seems to occur less frequently in circumcised males

Some studies suggest that circumcised males have fewer urine infections and fewer sexually transmitted diseases like syphilis and gonorrhea

Why People Don't Do It

The pain of the operation for the baby

Cultural tradition

Possible side effects such as bleeding, infection, or urinary problems

Personal beliefs, for example, that uncircumcised males have better sexual performance

No medical proof that a circumcised penis is easier to keep clean

Debate among professionals about whether circumcision protects a man from cancer of the penis or from sexually transmitted diseases

Flesch-Kincaid Reading Level: 7.8

Special Instructions _____

_____

_____

_____

Phone number to call if you have questions: _____

Copyright © Lippincott Williams & Wilkins. Developed by MC Freda, EdD, RN, CHES, FAAN.

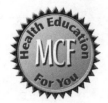

LA CIRCUNCISION ES SU DECISION

La circuncisión es una cirugía que se hace en bebés varones, en la cual la piel que cubre la cabeza del pene (llamada "prepucio") se remueve. La Academia Americana de Pedíatria (1999) ha indicado que no pueden recomendar la circuncisión rutinariamente porque no hay ninguna razón médica necesaria para hacerla. Sin embargo, mucha gente cree que la circuncisión es la cosa correcta de hacer. No hay respuestas claras. Se le pedirá que decida si desea que su recién nacido tenga una circuncisión. Esta página le dará información sobre algunas de las cosas que debe tener en cuenta. Asegúrese que hable con su doctor, partera, enfermera y pediatra también. Asegúrese también si su seguro cubre la circuncisión.

¿Porqué La Gente Lo Hacen?

La religión o tracidición cultural

La tradición familiar, tales como que el padre del niño o hermanos han tenido la circuncisión

Creencias personales, por ejemplo, la creencia que el pene circuncidado es más facil de mantener limpio o que los varones circuncisados tienen una mejor realización sexual

Si la circuncisión se hace más tarde en la vida es requerido que sea admitido al hospital

Algunos investigadores, sugieren que el cancer del pene, aunque sea una enfermedad rara, parece ocurrir menos frecuentemente en varones circuncisados

Algunos estudios sugieren que los varones circuncisados tienen menos infecciones de la orina, y menos enfermedades transmitidas sexualmente como el sífilis y la gonorrea

¿Porqué La Gente No Lo Hacen?

El dolor de la operación al bebé

La tradición cultural

Posibles efectos secundarios como sangramiento, infección o problemas urinarios

Creencias personales, por ejemplo, que los varones circuncisados tienen una mejor relación sexual

No hay prueba médica que indique el pene circuncidado es más facil de mantener limpio

El debate entre profecionales sobre si la circuncisión protege a los hombres contra el cáncer del pene o contra enfermedades transmitidas sexualmente

Special Instructions _____

_____

_____

Phone number to call if you have questions: _____

Copyright © Lippincott Williams & Wilkins. Developed by MC Freda, EdD, RN, CHES, FAAN.

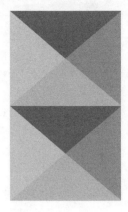

chapter 11

Postpartum Care

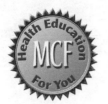

Woman's name: _____

Date: _____

Nurse's name: _____

After Your Baby Is Born

What happens to the baby right after birth?

In many hospitals, and probably in all birthing centers, a healthy baby stays with the family as long as the parents want. Some hospitals have rules that the baby has to go to a nursery for a few hours to be examined and weighed. Other hospitals leave the baby with you, and the examinations are done in your room. You should ask your doctor, nurse, or midwife what happens at the place you have chosen to give birth, and let him or her know what you want.

What happens to me? Do I go to another room or stay where I gave birth?

This depends on the type of setting you chose for the birth.

- In a birthing center you will probably stay in the room where you gave birth. At many birthing centers you stay there for 6 to 12 hours, and then go home, most of the time in 24 hours.
- In a hospital, there are different ways of doing things. Some hospitals have what are called "LDRP" rooms. That means Labor, Delivery, Recovery, and Postpartum. You would stay in the same room from the time you get admitted until you go home, usually 24 to 48 hours later.
- Some hospitals have just LDR rooms. After the "recovery" period—usually about 1 hour—you will be transferred to a postpartum room where you will stay until you go home.
- In some hospitals you labor in one room, give birth in a different room, have recovery in another room, and then go to the postpartum room.

If I'm in the hospital for 1 to 2 days after birth, where is the baby?

This also depends on the rules of the place you have chosen. In birthing centers, the baby will probably be with you all the time. In some hospitals the baby stays with you all the time also. In other hospitals, the baby is kept in a nursery, and brought out to you at feeding times. In other hospitals, the baby can stay with you during the day, but goes to the nursery at night.

You should know the rules in the place you'll be giving birth. Ask your doctor, nurse or midwife about this.

Flesch-Kincaid Reading Level: 6.0

Special Instructions _____

_____

Phone number to call if you have questions: _____

Copyright © Lippincott Williams & Wilkins. Developed by MC Freda, EdD, RN, CHES, FAAN.

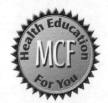

Woman's name: _____
Date: _____
Nurse's name: _____

Después del Nacimiento del Bebé

¿Qué le sucede al bebé después del nacimiento?

En muchos hospitals y probablemente en todos los centros de maternidad, un bebé saludable se puede quedar con su familia por el tiempo que los padres quieran. Algunos hospitals observan ciertas reglas; que el bebé debe de ir a la guardería por unas horas, para ser examinado y pesado. Otros hospitals dejan al bebé contigo y las pruebas son hechas en tu cuarto. Debes de preguntarle a tu doctor, enfermera o comadrona que es lo regular en el lugar que has escogido para el nacimeinto de tu bebé y déjale saber que es lo que tu deseas.

¿Qué me va a suceder? ¿Voy a otro cuarto, o me quedo donde dí a luz?

Esto depende del tipo de cuarto que hayas escogido:

- En un centro de maternidad probablemente te quedarás donde hayas dado a luz. En muchos centros te puedes quedar por 6-12 horas, y después te vas a casa, la mayoría de las veces te quedas por 24 horas.
- En un hospital, existen muchas opciones. Algunos hospitales tienen lo que se conoce como cuarto de "LDRP," esto incluye el parto, recuperación y postparto. Te quedarías en el mismo cuarto desde el momento de admisión hasta que te vayas a la casa, por lo general 24-48 horas.
- Algunos hospitales solamente tienen cuartos de parto y de recuperación. Después eres transferida a un cuarto de postparto donde te quedarás hasta que sea el momento de irte a casa
- En algunos hospitales pasas los dolores de parto en un cuarto, das a luz en otro cuarto, te recuperas en otro cuarto y después te vas al cuarto de postparto

Si yo estoy en el hospital por 1-2 días, ¿dónde se encuentra mi bebé?

Esto también depende de las reglas del sitio que hayas escogido para dar a luz. En centros de maternidad, el bebé generalmente estará contigo todo el tiempo. En algunos hospitales el bebé también se queda contigo todo el tiempo. En otros hospitales, el bebé se queda en la guardería, y te lo traen cuando sea hora de comer. En otro hospitales, el bebé se queda contigo todo el día, pero se va a la guardería por la noche.

Deberías de informarte sobre las reglas del lugar donde vas a dar a luz. Pregúntale a tu doctor, enfermera o comadrona sobre este asunto.

Special Instructions _____

_____

Phone number to call if you have questions: _____

Copyright © Lippincott Williams & Wilkins. Developed by MC Freda, EdD, RN, CHES, FAAN.

Woman's name: _____

Date: _____

Nurse's name: _____

Understanding Your Feelings After Having a Baby

What are the "Baby Blues?"

Many women feel "blue" or sad during the first few weeks after childbirth. Some women find themselves crying for no reason, feel very tired, have trouble sleeping (and not just because the baby is awake), have trouble concentrating, or feel angry or irritable. These are symptoms of the Baby Blues. This can last about a week. There really isn't anything you can do about it, because it's a reaction to all the hormone changes in your body, but if you understand what's happening it doesn't seem so frightening.

How do I know if I have something more serious than Baby Blues?

Unfortunately, some women get something worse after having a baby called "Postpartum Depression." Postpartum depression is very different from Baby Blues. It is a serious illness that usually starts about 1 month after the baby is born and can last from 3 to 12 months. Women who have postpartum depression feel much more than "blue." Some women have said they feel like everything is falling apart or like they are losing their minds. Some women even say they feel like hurting themselves or their babies.

What are the symptoms of postpartum depression?

You don't need to have all of these symptoms, but these are the most common:

Crying	Unable to sleep	Change in appetite
Feeling worthless	No energy	Can't concentrate
Feeling anxious	Don't care about the way you look	
Feeling hostile	Feeling irritable most of the time	

What do I do if I think I have postpartum depression?

If you feel any of the symptoms and can't seem to feel better, you need to call your doctor, nurse, or midwife. These feelings are not your fault. You didn't make them happen. This is a sickness that needs to be treated. Don't be afraid to call for help.

Flesch-Kincaid Reading Level: 6.3

Special Instructions _____

_____

_____

_____

Phone number to call if you have questions: _____

Copyright © Lippincott Williams & Wilkins. Developed by MC Freda, EdD, RN, CHES, FAAN.

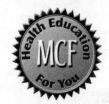

Woman's name: _____
Date: _____
Nurse's name: _____

Entendiendo tus Emociones Después el Parto

¿Qué es "Baby Blues"?

Muchas mujeres se sienten tristes o melancólicas durante las primeras semanas después del parto. Algunas mujeres sienten ganas de llorar sin ninguna razón, se sienten muy cansadas, tienen problemas de dormir (y no es porque el bebé está despierto), tienen problemas de concentración, sienten rabia o irritabilidad. Estos son síntomas de lo que se conoce como "Baby Blues". Esto puede durar cerca de una semana. En realidad no hay nada que se pueda hacer al respecto, ya que es una reacción normal de los cambios hormonales del cuerpo. Sin embargo, si entiendes mejor que es lo que te está sucediendo, no te parecería tan alarmante.

¿Cómo sé si tengo algo más grave que "Baby Blue"?

Desafortunadamente, algunas mujeres sufren de algo más grave después del parto, conocido como "Depresión del Postparto". Depresión del Postparto es algo muy diferente a "Baby Blue". Es una enfermedad muy grave la cual comienza alrededor del primer mes después de nacido el bebé, y puede durar de tres a doce meses. Las mujeres que sufren de depresión del postparto sienten mucho más que tristeza. Muchas mujeres admiten que sienten que todo se les viene encima o que están perdiendo la razón, inclusive sienten el deseo de herirse así misma o al bebé.

¿Cuáles son los síntomas de la depresión del Postparto?

No necesitas sentir todos los síntomas juntos, pero éstos son los más comunes:

Llorar	No dormir	Cambio en el apetito
No autoestima	Falta de energía	No concentración
Ansiedad.	No importar la forma que luces	
Hostilidad	Irritable (la mayoría del tiempo)	

¿Qué puedo hacer si pienso que tengo Depresión del Postparto?

Si experimentas cualquiera de estos sintomas y pareciera que nunca te vas a curar, necesitas llamar de inmediato a tu doctor, enfermera o comadrona. Esta es una enfermedad que necesita tratamiento. No sientas miedo de pedir ayuda.

Special Instructions _____

_____

_____

Phone number to call if you have questions: _____

Copyright © Lippincott Williams & Wilkins. Developed by MC Freda, EdD, RN, CHES, FAAN.

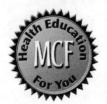

Woman's name: _____

Date: _____

Nurse's name: _____

Now That You've Decided to Breast-Feed . . .

Now that you've decided to breast-feed, you already know its many advantages. Your baby will get the best nutrition, as well as immunity to many diseases. Breast-feeding is low cost, is convenient, and also helps you get back into shape more quickly. So you've made a great decision!

What you might not know is that, although some women have no problems at all with breast-feeding, some women do experience problems in the beginning and need more help. If you are concerned about some aspect of breast-feeding, don't be afraid to call your doctor, nurse, or midwife. They know that breast-feeding can be difficult in the beginning for some women and they should be able to guide you. What's most important, however, is that you keep breast-feeding and not give up at the first sign of difficulty!

Helping you to learn about breast-feeding takes much more than this one sheet of paper. You can get lots of educational materials from the LaLeche League, a group of volunteers who help women breast-feed. Its number is (800) 525-3243. This handout is merely to help introduce you to some of the issues that might come up and to encourage you to speak to your provider, or to the LaLeche League, or to a lactation consultant (also in telephone books in some communities) if you have questions. Lactation consultants usually charge a fee for their services, so be sure to ask about that.

Here are some things to remember:

- You will probably have more uterine cramping when you breast-feed. This is good, and means that your uterus is going back to shape.
- One of the keys to effective breast-feeding is the way the baby latches on to the breast. The baby's mouth needs to cover the nipple and the dark areola.
- Breast-feeding should not hurt your nipple or breast. If it hurts, the baby might not be latched on properly. Don't let this stop you from breast-feeding. A lactation consultant or a LaLeche League person could help you if this is a problem.
- You should wear a nursing bra to support your breasts. If you have any leaking, buy nursing pads and put them in the bra.
- Most newborns breast-feed often for the first few weeks. Even if the baby is sleeping, don't go more than 5 to 6 hours without feeding.
- Sometimes your nipples might feel sore. Let them dry well before you put your bra back on after each feeding, and this should go away.

If you have any concerns, call your doctor, nurse or midwife.

Flesch-Kincaid Reading Level: 6.4

Special Instructions _____

_____

Phone number to call if you have questions: _____

Copyright © Lippincott Williams & Wilkins. Developed by MC Freda, EdD, RN, CHES, FAAN.

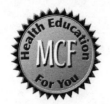

Woman's name: _____

Date: _____

Nurse's name: _____

Ahora que Ud Ha Decidido Amamantar . . .

Ahora que usted ha decidido amamantar, ya tiene conocimento de las ventajas que trae.

Su bebé obtendrá la mejor nutrición, así como tambien immunidad contra muchas enfermedades. El amamantar tiene bajo costo, es conveniente, y tambien le ayuda a que se ponga en forma mas rápidamente. Así que usted ha tomado una gran decisión!!!!

Lo que quizás usted no sabía es que mientras algunas mujeres no tienen ningún tipo de problema en amamantar a sus bebés, algunas mujeres experimentan problemas al principio, por lo que necesitan más ayuda. Si usted está preocupada por algunos de los aspectos del amamantar, no tenga miedo de llamar a su doctor, comadrona o enfermera. Ellos comprenden que el amamantar puede ser dificultoso al principio para algunas mujeres, así pués ellos estarán dispuestos a orientarles. De cualquier manera, lo importante es que usted siga amamantando a su bebé y no se rinda ante la primera señal de dificultad!

Usted necesita más que ésta hoja de papel para ayudarle a comprender sobre como amamantar a su bebé. Usted puede obtener muchos materiales educativos en La Liga de la Leche, éste es un grupo de voluntarios que orientan a las mujeres como amamantar a sus bebés. Su número es el (800) 525-3243. Este folleto es solamente para darle a conocer algunos de los temas de que se le puedan presentar y para estimularlos a que hablen con su proveedor, ó La Liga de la Leche, o un consultante de lactación (usted también puede encontrar a éstos consultantes en las guías telefónicas de algunas communidades). Usualmente éstos Consultantes de Lactacion cobran honoraios por su servicios, así que asegúrese de preguntar sobre el respecto.

He aquí algunos puntos para recordar:

- Muy probablemente usted sentirá más calambres uterinos cuando esté amamantando. Esto es bueno ya que su útero esta volviendo a su forma original.
- Una de las claves efectivas para un buen amamantamiento es la manera en que el bebé se prende del pecho de la madre. La boca del bebé necesita cubrir el pezón y la parte obscura del seno.
- El amamantar no implica dolor en el pecho o en el pezón. Si siente dolor, quiere decir que su bebé no está adecuadamente prendido de su pecho. No deje que ésto le impida amamantar a su bebé. Si ésto se convierte en un problema, consulte con un representate de La Liga de la Leche o con un consultante de Lactación.
- Use sostenes de maternidad como soporte a sus senos. Si éstos gotean leche, compre toallitas absorbentes e insértelas dentro del sostén. La mayoría de los recién nacidos amamantan cada una o dos horas durante las primeras semanas. Aunque el bebé esté durmiendo, no pase más de cinco o seis horas sin alimentarlo.
- Algunas veces sus pezones se sentirán adoloridos. Después de cada alimento, deje que sus pezones se sequen completamente antes de ponerse su sostén. De esta forma se sentirán menos adoloridos.

Si tiene alguna pregunta, llame a sus doctor, enfermera o comadrona.

Special Instructions _____

_____

Phone number to call if you have questions: _____

Copyright © Lippincott Williams & Wilkins. Developed by MC Freda, EdD, RN, CHES, FAAN.

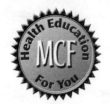

Woman's name: _____
Date: _____
Nurse's name: _____

How Your Body Heals After Childbirth

Bleeding

In the first few days after you give birth, you will probably start to have cramps in your abdomen. This means that your uterus is starting to shrink back to its former shape. You will also have bleeding from your vagina, like a heavy period. This is called "lochia" (pronounced "low-key-ah") and is usually dark red, might have clots in it, or is sometimes brown. Around the 3rd or 4th day, this discharge turns a lighter pink and stays like that until about 2 weeks after the baby is born. Then the discharge becomes yellow or white and can last several more weeks.

Emotions

Most women feel a mixture of emotions after they give birth. They often feel excited and exhausted, happy and tearful, tired yet full of energy. Some women want to be alone with their baby, some want to have all their loved ones around them. The important thing to remember is that there are no rulebooks to tell you how you should feel. Whatever you are feeling is right for you. It's true, however, that what most women want after going through labor is some rest! The amount of energy you use in labor has been compared to running a marathon, so you deserve as much rest as you want.

What about sex?

Most women wonder when they can have sex after childbirth. Most women are comfortable having sex again after the vaginal discharge has stopped, which is about 1 month after giving birth. If you had stitches, you might need a few weeks for it to heal before you have sex. Speak to your doctor, nurse, or midwife about this.

If any of these things happen during the first few weeks after birth, you need to call your doctor, nurse or midwife:

- You have a fever or severe pain
- You begin to bleed a lot of red blood again after it had changed to pink
- Your vaginal discharge has an odor (this could mean an infection)
- You start to have large blood clots in the discharge
- If you had stitches, any sharp pain near them that doesn't go away could mean an infection

Flesch-Kincaid Reading Level: 5.9

Special Instructions _____

_____

Phone number to call if you have questions: _____

Copyright © Lippincott Williams & Wilkins. Developed by MC Freda, EdD, RN, CHES, FAAN.

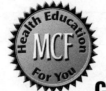

Como tu Cuerpo se Recupera Después del Parto

Sangramiento

En los primeros días después del parto, quizás comenzarás a sentir calambres en tu abdomen. Esto indica que el útero está regresando a su forma y tamaño normal. También sangrarás por tu vagina, como un periodo abundante. Esto se llama "loquia", y por lo general es de color rojo obscuro con mucho coágulos, a veces es de color marrón. Alrededor del 3ro o 4to día, éste flujo se transforma en rosado claro y se queda así por lo menos 2 semanas después que el bebé nazca. Luego éste flujo se vuelve amarillo o blanco, y puede durar así un par de semanas más.

Emociones

Muchas mujeres experimentan una mezcla de emociones después del parto. Por lo general se sienten excitadas y agotadas, felices y llorosas, cansadas pero con mucha energía. Algunas mujeres quieren estar solas con sus bebés, otras quieren estar rodeadas de sus seres queridos. Es importante recordar que no hay ninguna regla que diga cómo debes sentirte. Sea lo que estés sintiendo, es bueno para tí. Sin embargo, es verdad que lo que muchas mujeres desean después del parto es descanso!!! La cantidad de energía utilizada durante un parto se compara al correr un maratón, así que mereces descansar todo lo que quieras.

¿Y sobre el sexo?

Muchas mujeres se preguntan cuando pueden tener sexo después del parto. La mayoría de las mujeres se sienten confortables con la idea de tener sexo después que el flujo vaginal ha parado, lo cual sucede alrededor del primer mes después del nacimiento. Si te han dado puntos, necesitarías unas cuantas semanas más para curarte y resumir el sexo. Consulta con tu doctor, enfermera o comadrona sobre ésto.

Si cualquier de estos señales suceden durante las primeras semanas después del parto, necesitas llamar a un doctor, enfermera o comadrona:

- Tienes fiebre ó dolor intenso.
- Comienzas a sangrar abundantemente después que la sangre había cambiado de rojo a rosado.
- El flujo vaginal tiene mal olor(ésto significa una infección)
- Comienzan a salir coágulos grandes en el flujo.
- Si te han dado puntos, cualquier dolor puntiagudo cerca de ellos podría significar una infección.

Special Instructions _____

_____

Phone number to call if you have questions: _____

Copyright © Lippincott Williams & Wilkins. Developed by MC Freda, EdD, RN, CHES, FAAN.

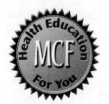

Woman's name: _____

Date: _____

Nurse's name: _____

Healing After a Cesarean Birth

Women who have a cesarean birth need some extra time for healing because they had abdominal surgery. You will probably stay in the hospital a few days longer than women with a vaginal birth, but each hospital has its own rules about that, so check with your doctor, nurse, or midwife.

What about the stitches?

There are two types of stitches. The stitches on the inside will dissolve while you heal, and they do not have to be removed. The stitches (or staples) on the outside have to be removed. That usually happens about 7 days after the cesarean, but your doctor will tell you when to have that done. While the outside staples or stitches are still in, you should keep that area clean, with a clean and dry bandage over it.

How will I know if anything is wrong?

- If you have a fever, or a lot of pain or redness or swelling at your incision, or if there is any fluid or pus coming out of your incision, you should call your doctor, because you could have an infection.
- Another complication could be a blood clot in the lower leg, so if you have pain in your calf muscle, or your lower leg feels hot, call your doctor.
- If you feel extremely sad, or feel that you can't be a good mother to your baby, and that feeling doesn't go away after about one week, you need to call your doctor, because you could be suffering from postpartum depression. This can be treated, so it's important to tell your doctor about it.

What about gas pains?

Many women who have cesarean birth have gas pains, and they can really hurt! The best thing to do is to drink a lot of water (8 glasses each day), walk as much as you can, and eat fruits and vegetables. If you become constipated, call your doctor for medication to help you.

How long will it take for me to feel like myself again?

Some women need about 6 weeks to feel like themselves again after a cesarean birth. Some women feel better sooner. Remember that you had a major surgery, so your body needs time to get better. Be sure to rest whenever you can, drink a lot of fluids, and eat healthy foods, and you'll soon be back to normal.

Flesch-Kincaid Reading Level: 6.7

Special Instructions _____

Phone number to call if you have questions: _____

Copyright © Lippincott Williams & Wilkins. Developed by MC Freda, EdD, RN, CHES, FAAN.

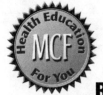

Woman's name: _____

Date: _____

Nurse's name: _____

Recuperación Después de un Parto por Cesárea

Las mujeres que han tenido un parto por cesárea necesitan más tiempo para sanarse, ya que fueron sometidas a un cirugía abdominal. Probablemente se quedará en el hospital por unos días más que una mujer que tuvo un parto normal o vaginal, pero cada hospital tienen sus reglas sobre ésto, así que hable con su doctor, enfermera o comadrona.

¿Qué hacer sobre los puntos?

Hay dos tipos de puntos. Los puntos internos se disolverán mientras te curas, y no tienen que ser removidos. Los puntos (o grapas) en la parte de afuera tienen que ser removidos. Esto pasa generalmente alrededor de los 7 días después de la cesárea, pero tu doctor te dirá cuando se le removeran los puntos. Mientras tengan los puntos ó grapas, mantenga esa área limpia, con un bendaje limpio y seco sobre la herida.

¿Cómo sabré si algo anda mal?

- Si tienes fiebre o mucho dolor o enrojecimiento o hinchazón en la herida o si hay líquido o pus saliendo de la herida, llame a su doctor, porque pudiera tener una infección
- Otra complicación puede ser un coágulo de sangre en la parte baja de la pierna, así que si tienes dolor en la pantorrilla o si tus piernas se sienten caliente, llame a su doctor
- Si te sientes exrtremadamente triste o sientes que no puedes ser una buena madre para tu niño, y si estos sentimientos no se alivian por más de una semana, necesitas llamar a tu doctor, porque podrías estar sufriendo de depresión del postparto. Esto puede ser tratado, así que es muy importante hablar con tu doctor sobre ello.

¿Dolores por los Gases?

Muchas mujeres que han tenido parto por cesárea sufren de dolores a causa de los gases, y éstos pueden ser bien dolorosos!!! Lo mejor que puedes hacer es tomar mucho agua (8 vasos diarios) caminar cuanto puedas, y comer muchas frutas y vegetales. Si te extriñes, llama a tu doctor para que te recete algún medicamento que la ayude

¿Cuánto tiempo me tomará para sentirme como antes?

Algunas mujeres necesitan de 6 semanas para recuperarse por completo después de un parto por cesárea. Otras se sienten bien en menos tiempo. Recuerda que has tenido una operación mayor, así que tu cuerpo necesita tiempo para sentirse mejor. Asegúrate de descansar cuanto puedas, toma mucho líquidos, come nutritivamente, y pronto estarás normal como antes.

Special Instructions _____

Phone number to call if you have questions: _____

Copyright © Lippincott Williams & Wilkins. Developed by MC Freda, EdD, RN, CHES, FAAN.

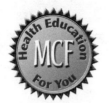

Woman's name: _____

Date: _____

Nurse's name: _____

Kegel Exercises

"Kegel exercises" are special exercises that you need to do to make the muscles near your bladder and vagina stronger. If you are pregnant, this can help you get ready for the birth of your baby and can make you feel better after the baby is born. If you are not pregnant, Kegel exercises can keep that part of your body in shape.

This is how you find the right muscles

- You can't see these muscles. You need to feel them. One way is to pretend that you are trying to hold something in your vagina. Tighten those muscles for a few seconds.
- Another way to feel those muscles is to try to start and then quickly stop your urine when you are going to the bathroom. When you try to stop, then you are using those muscles.

This is how you do the Kegel Exercises

- Think about the muscles you need to use, then squeeze them tightly.
- Hold the muscles tightly for 2 seconds, then let them go.
- Do this 10 times in a row the first day.
- Every day do this 10 more times than the last day, until you are doing it for 5 minutes every day.

You can do these exercises any time at all. You can do them when you are home alone, when you are sitting in a car or a bus, when you are talking on the phone, or at other times.

Talk to your doctor, nurse, or midwife for more information about this.

Flesch-Kincaid Reading Level: 4.5

Special Instructions _____

_____

_____

_____

_____

Phone number to call if you have questions: _____

Copyright © Lippincott Williams & Wilkins. Developed by MC Freda, EdD, RN, CHES, FAAN.

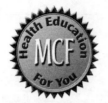

Woman's name: _____

Date: _____

Nurse's name: _____

Ejercicios Kegel

Los "Ejercicios Kegel" son ejercicios especiales que debe hacer para que los músculos cerca de su vejiga y vagina estén fuertes. Si está embarazada, esto la puede ayudar a estar lista para el nacimiento de su bebé y la puede hacer sentir mejor después que su bebé nazca. Si no está embarazada, los Ejercicios Kegel pueden manterner esa parte de su cuerpo en forma.

Aquí le diremos como encontrar los músculos correctos:

- No puede ver estos músculos. Necesita sentirlos. Una manera es pretender que está sosteniendo algo en su vagina. Oprima estos músculos por unos cuantos segundos.
- Otra manera de sentir estos músculos es tratar de comenzar y después rápidamente parar su orina cuando esté en el baño. Cuando trate de parar entonces estará usando estos músculos.

Aquí le diremos como hacer los Ejercicios Kegel:

- Piense en los músculos que necesita usar y después aprietelos fuertemente.
- Mantenga los músculos fuertemente por 2 segundos, y después sueltelos.
- Haga esto 10 veces seguidas el primer día.
- Todos los días haga esto 10 veces más cada día, hasta que lo haga por 5 minutos cada día.

Puede hacer estos ejercicios en cualquier momento. Los puede hacer mientras esté en casa sola, o mientras esté sentada en un carro o bus, mientras esté hablando por teléfono, o en otros momentos.

Hable con su doctor, enfermera o partera para obtener más información sobre esto.

Special Instructions _____

_____

_____

_____

_____

_____

Phone number to call if you have questions: _____

Copyright © Lippincott Williams & Wilkins. Developed by MC Freda, EdD, RN, CHES, FAAN.

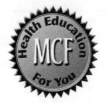

Woman's name: _____

Date: _____

Nurse's name: _____

Do You Know About "Back to Sleep"???

Have you heard about Back to Sleep? This is one of the most important things you should know about taking care of a newborn baby. Back to Sleep means putting your baby to bed on his or her back, all the time.

We now know that putting babies to bed on their backs can prevent Sudden Infant Death Syndrome (SIDS), which is the leading cause of death for infants between 1 month and 1 year of age. It's amazing, but a simple thing like putting a baby to bed on his or her back can make a big difference. Since 1992, doctors and nurses have been giving this advice to parents, and deaths due to SIDS have dropped by 42%.

Some people don't understand how important this is and might tell you (because they were told many years ago) that babies should only be put to sleep on their tummies, but please don't listen to them! It is safe to put babies to bed on their backs, and the drop in number of cases of SIDS is real.

Ask your doctor, nurse or midwife about this. They'll tell you:

BACK TO SLEEP!!!!!

Flesch-Kincaid Reading Level: 5.3

Special Instructions _____

_____

_____

_____

_____

_____

_____

Phone number to call if you have questions: _____

Copyright © Lippincott Williams & Wilkins. Developed by MC Freda, EdD, RN, CHES, FAAN.

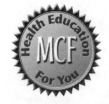

Woman's name: _____

Date: _____

Nurse's name: _____

¿Sabe Usted lo que es "Dormir de Espalda"?

¿Has escuchado alguna vez del dicho "Dormir de Espalda"? Este es un factor muy importante que deberías saber sobre el cuidado de un recién nacido. "Dormir de Espalda" significa poner a dormir a su bebé de espalda en la cama, a toda hora.

Sabemos que poniendo a dormir de espalda a los infantes puede prevenir el Síndrome Súbita de Muerte Infantil, el cual es la causa principal de muerte en infantes de 1 mes a 1 año de edad. Es increíble, pero el simple hecho de poner a su bebé de espalda a la hora de dormir hace una gran diferencia. Desde 1992, doctores y enfermeras han aconsejando a los padres sobre ésto, y el índice de muerte por el Síndrome, ha disminuído en un 42%.

Algunas personas no entienden lo importante que ésto es, inclusive te podrían decir (porque les fueron aconsejados muchos años atrás) que los bebés deben de dormir de estómago, pero por favor no les presten atención! Es seguro poner a dormir a su bebé de espalda y la baja en el número de incidentes por el síndrome son reales.

Pregunte a su doctor, enfermera o comadrona sobre este asunto. Ellos le dirán:

"DORMIR DE ESPALDA"

Special Instructions _____

_____

_____

_____

_____

_____

_____

Phone number to call if you have questions: _____

Copyright © Lippincott Williams & Wilkins. Developed by MC Freda, EdD, RN, CHES, FAAN.

Woman's name: _____

Date: _____

Nurse's name: _____

Some Things You Need to Know About Taking the Birth Control Pill

How to Take The Pill

- Take a pill every day. When one pack is finished, start a new pack.
- Remember that pills don't protect you from diseases such as AIDS and STDs—use condoms.
- There are a few different types of pills. Ask your doctor, nurse, or midwife exactly what type you are being given and write the name down here:

  The name of the pill you have been given is _____.

  _____Yours is a "Day One" pill. Take the first pill on the first day of your period.

  _____Yours is a "Sunday start" pill. Take the first pill on the first Sunday after your period begins. Take the pill even if you are still bleeding on that Sunday. If your period begins on a Sunday, take the pill that day.

When Is the Best Time to Take the Pill?

Some people take the pill before going to bed, or first thing in the morning. **It doesn't matter what time you take it—the only important thing is that you take the pill at the same time every single day.**

Are You Protected Right Away From Getting Pregnant?

During the first 2 weeks you take the pills, you could still get pregnant, so use condoms. You should be protected from getting pregnant after that.

What to Do If You Make a Mistake With Your Pills

If you forget to take a pill at your usual time, take one as soon as you remember.

If you forget to take a pill for 1 whole day, take 2 pills the next day.

Be sure to use condoms if you forget to take your pills.

If you forget to take pills on 2 days, you are no longer protected from getting pregnant. You will have to start with a new month of pills after your next period.

What to Do If You Have No Period

Continue taking the pills, but call your doctor, nurse, or midwife and ask what to do next.

What to Do If You Spot or Stain While Taking The Pill

This happens sometimes. Don't be worried. If the spotting doesn't stop after 2 packs of pills, then call your doctor, nurse, or midwife.

Flesch-Kincaid Reading Level: 4.6

Special Instructions _____

_____

_____

Phone number to call if you have questions: _____

Copyright © Lippincott Williams & Wilkins. Developed by MC Freda, EdD, RN, CHES, FAAN.

MCF
Health Education For You

Algo Que Debe Saber Acerca De Tomar Pastillas Anticonceptivas

Como tomar la pastilla

- Tome una pastilla diaria. Cuando un paquete termine, inicie otro.
- Recuerde, las pastillas no la protegen de enfermedades como el SIDA y los ETS, use condones.
- Hay diferentes tipos de pastillas. Pregúntele a su doctor, enfermera o partera que tipo se le ha dado y escriba el nombre debajo:

    El nombre de la pastilla que se le ha dado es _____

    _____La suya es la pastilla del "primer día". Tome la primera el primer día de su periodo.

    _____La suya es la pastilla de "Inicio Domingo". Tome la primera pastilla el primer domingo después que su periodo ha comenzado. Tómela aún si está sangrando ese domingo. Si su periodo empieza un domingo tome la pastilla ese día

¿Cuándo es el mejor tiempo de tomar la pastilla?

Algunas personas toman la pastilla antes de acostarse, o temprano al levantarse. No importa la hora en que la tome - Lo importante es que la tome a la misma hora todos los días.

¿Está protegida del embarazo inmediatamente?

Durante las pimeras dos semanas de estar tamando la pastilla, podría quedar embarazada, por eso, use condones. Después de ésto ya debe estar protegida.

¿Qué Hacer Si Comete Un Error Con Sus Pastillas?

Si se olvida de tomar la pastilla a la hora usual, tome una tan pronto se acuerde

Si se olvida de tomar la pastilla por un día completo, tome 2 el próximo día

Asegurase de usar condones si se olvida de tomar la pastilla

Si se olvida de tomar la pastilla por 2 días, ya no está protegida

Tendrías que iniciar un nuevo mes de pastilla en su próximo periodo

¿Qué hacer si no tiene su periodo?

Continue tomando las pastillas, pero llame a su doctor, enfermera ó partera y pregunta que debe hacer.

¿Qué Hacer Si Mancha Mientras Tome las Pastillas?

Esto pasa a veces. No se preocupe. Si el manchado no para después de 2 paquetes de pastillas, llame a su doctor, enfermera o partera.

Special Instructions _____

_____

_____

Phone number to call if you have questions: _____

Copyright © Lippincott Williams & Wilkins. Developed by MC Freda, EdD, RN, CHES, FAAN.

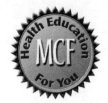

Woman's name: _____

Date: _____

Nurse's name: _____

Depo-Provera

What Is It??? How Does It Work???

Depo-Provera, the birth control "shot," is an injection of the female hormone Progesterone. People call it different names: "Depo-Provera," "DMPA," or sometimes just "the shot." When you choose Depo-Provera for birth control, you get one shot every 3 months. It works by stopping eggs from being released from the ovaries. Your period changes after you have had the Depo-Provera shot for birth control. Most women have fewer periods the longer they use Depo-Provera.

Advantages of Using Depo-Provera for Birth Control

It prevents pregnancy 99% of the time

It usually decreases the bleeding and cramps during your period

It can be used by women who are breast-feeding

You don't have to think about birth control every day, or when you have sex

> *Depo-Provera Cannot Protect You From AIDS Or Any Other Sexually Transmitted Disease. You Must Use Condoms For That.*

Disadvantages of Using Depo-Provera

Some, but not all, women who use Depo-Provera have complained of:

Spotting, occasional heavy vaginal bleeding, or no period at all

Feeling depressed

Increased appetite and weight gain

Acne or oily skin

Allergic reactions

Not being able to get pregnant for 6 to 12 months after stopping the shots

If you decide to get Depo-Provera it is important that you have regular check-ups when you are using it for birth control. Be sure to ask your doctor, nurse, or midwife any questions you have about Depo-Provera.

Flesch-Kincaid Reading Level: 7.0

Special Instructions _____

_____

_____

Phone number to call if you have questions: _____

Copyright © Lippincott Williams & Wilkins. Developed by MC Freda, EdD, RN, CHES, FAAN.

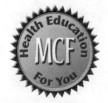

Woman's name: _____

Date: _____

Nurse's name: _____

DEPO-PROVERA

¿¿¿Qué Es??? ¿¿¿Cómo Funciona???

Depo-Provera, la "inyección" de prevención del embarazo, es una inyección de la hormona femenina Progesterona. Tiene diferentes nombres: "Depo-Provera", "DMPA," o algunas veces "la inyección." Cuando decide usar Depo-Provera para prevenir el embarazo, se da una inyección cada tres meses. Funciona al parar que los huevos sean soltados de los ovarios. Su periodo cambia después que se le dé la inyección de Depo-Provera de prevención del embarazo. La mayoría de las mujeres tienen menos periodos cuanto más usen "la inyección."

Ventajas Del Uso De Depo-Provera Para Prevenir El Embarazo

Previene el embarazo 99% del tiempo

Normalmente disminuye el sangramiento y calambre abdominal durante su periodo

Puede ser usado por mujeres que esten dando de mamar

No tiene que pensar sobre prevención del embarazo todos los días ó cuando tiene relaciones sexuales

> **Depo-Provera No La Puede Proteger Contra**
> **El SIDA U Otras Enfermedades Transmitidas Sexualmente.**
> **Tiene Que Usar Condones Para Eso.**

Desventajas Del Uso de Depo-Provera

Algunas, pero no todas, las mujeres que usan Depo-Provera se han quejado de:

De estar Manchando, de un fuerte sangramiento vaginal, o falta de periodo por completo

Sentirse deprimida

Aumento de apetito y de peso

Acne o piel grasosa

Reacciones alérgicas

No poder embarazarse de 6 a 12 meses después de parar las inyecciones

Si decide recibir el Depo-Provera es importante que tenga chequeos regulares mientras esté usándolo para prevenir el embarazo. Asegúrese de preguntar a su doctor, enfermera o partera si tiene alguna pregunta sobre el Depo-Provera.

Special Instructions _____

Phone number to call if you have questions: _____

Copyright © Lippincott Williams & Wilkins. Developed by MC Freda, EdD, RN, CHES, FAAN.

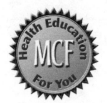

Woman's name: _____

Date: _____

Nurse's name: _____

What Every Woman Should Know About Foam and Condoms

Condoms are the only way to protect yourself from Sexually Transmitted Diseases (STDs) such as Syphilis, Gonorrhea, Chlamydia, and AIDS.

Do You Really Know How to Use Condoms???

You might think you know how to use condoms, but if you use them wrong, then it's like not using them at all. Condoms, which are used to cover the penis, should be used with **"foam,"** which kills sperm. If you use condoms and foam every time you have sex, and if you use them the right way, you can feel fairly safe about protecting yourself not only from pregnancy, but also from STDs.

Here Is the Right Way to Use Condoms and Foam

- Push the foam applicator over the foam container and fill the applicator
- Put the foam into your vagina like you would use a tampon, but **no more than 30 minutes before you have sex**
- Wash the applicator with soap and water after each use
- Take the condom out of the package and roll it onto the penis after the penis is hard but **before** it is close to the vagina
- Leave 1/2 inch of space at the tip of the penis—this gives the sperm a place to go
- After sex, take the penis out **while holding the condom on the penis**
- If the condom breaks, quickly insert more foam, **but if you don't get a regular period the next month, be sure to get a pregnancy test**
- Never use a condom more than once
- Never use Vaseline or cold cream in your vagina or on the penis—they can make the condom break

Always keep extra foam and condoms around. Talk to your doctor, nurse, or midwife if you have questions about this.

Flesch-Kincaid Reading Level: 6.2

Special Instructions _____

_____

_____

_____

Phone number to call if you have questions: _____

Copyright © Lippincott Williams & Wilkins. Developed by MC Freda, EdD, RN, CHES, FAAN.

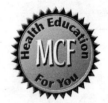

Woman's name: _____

Date: _____

Nurse's name: _____

Lo Que Toda Mujer Debe Saber Acerca De La Espuma Y Condones

Los condones son la única forma para protegerse de Enfermedades Transmitidas Sexualmente (ETS) tales como Sífilis, Gonorrea, Clamidia Y SIDA.

¿¿Realmente Sabe Como Usar Condones??

Podría pensar que sabe como usar condones, pero si los usa incorrectamente, es como si no los usara. Los condones que son usados para cubrir el pene, deben ser usados con la "espuma", la cual mata el esperma. Si usas condón y la espuma siempre que tengas sexo, y si los usas correctamente, puede sentirse segura que está protegida del embarazo y de ETS también.

Esta Es La Forma Correcta De Usar Condones Y La Espuma:

- Empuje el aplicador de la espuma sobre el recipiente de espuma y llene el aplicador
- Ponga la espuma en su vagina como si aplicaría un tapón sanitario, **pero no más de 30 minutos antes de tener sexo**
- Lave el aplicador con jabón y agua después de cada uso
- Saque el condón de la envoltura y coloque el pene dentro cuando esté firme, pero antes que esté cerca de la vagina
- Deje un espacio de 1/2 pulgada en la punta del pene—esto le da un espacio al esperma para depositarse después del sexo, saque el pene **con el condón puesto**
- Si se rompe el condón, rápidamente apliquese más espuma, **pero si no ve su periodo regular el próximo mes, asegúrese de hacerse una prueba de embarazo**
- Nunca use un condón más de una vez
- Nunca use vaselina o crema fría en su vagina o en le pene—esto puede hacer romper el condón

Siempre mantenga extra espuma y condones a su alcance hable con su doctor, enfermera o partera si tiene preguntas al respecto

Special Instructions _____

_____

_____

_____

Phone number to call if you have questions: _____

Copyright © Lippincott Williams & Wilkins. Developed by MC Freda, EdD, RN, CHES, FAAN.

MCF · Health Education · For You

Are You Thinking About Tubal Sterilization?????

"Tubal Sterilization" is called many different things. Some people call it "tubal ligation," or "tubal cutting," or "tubal burning," or "having your tubes tied." They all mean the same thing.

This is a very important family planning decision. We want to be sure you understand exactly what "tubal sterilization" is all about. When you have this operation done, you are deciding that you will **never** have any more pregnancies. Some women think they can have their tubes "tied," or "cut," or "burned," and then have another operation to change them back and become pregnant again. That is not possible for most women. A tubal sterilization is permanent. Unless you are 100% sure that you never want another pregnancy, then choose a different form of birth control. Ask your doctor, nurse, or midwife about this.

Tubal sterilization is usually done as an operation, after your baby is born. If you decide to have tubal sterilization, you have to sign special consent papers saying that you understand you will never have another pregnancy.

Flesch-Kincaid Reading Level: 7.3

Special Instructions _____

_____

_____

_____

_____

_____

_____

Phone number to call if you have questions: _____

Copyright © Lippincott Williams & Wilkins. Developed by MC Freda, EdD, RN, CHES, FAAN.

¿¿¿Está Pensando En La Esterilización Tubal?????

La "Esterilización tubal" es llamada de diferente maneras. Algunos la llaman "Ligación De Tubo", "Cortarse El Tubo" o "Quemarse El Tubo". Todos estos nombres significan lo mismo.

Esta es una decisión muy importante de planeameinto de familia. Queremos estar seguros que entienda exactamente lo que la "esterilización tubal" es. Al hacerse esta operación , está decidiendo que **nunca** más prodrá tener más embarazos. Algunas mujeres piensan que pueden "ligarse", "cortarse" o "quemarse" los tubos y luego operarse de nuevo y volver a quedar embarazadas. Esto no es posible para la mayoría de las mujeres. La esterilización de tubos es permanente. Si no está 100% segura de nunca más querer otro embarazo entonces escoga otra forma de control del embarazo. Pregúntele a su doctor, enfermera o partera sobre esto.

La esterilización tubal es usualmente hecho como una operación, después del nacimiento de su bebé. Si decide hacerse la esterilización tubal, debe firmar un papel de consentimiento que aclara que entiende que nunca más tendrá otro embarazo.

Special Instructions _____

_____

_____

_____

_____

_____

_____

Phone number to call if you have questions: _____

Copyright © Lippincott Williams & Wilkins. Developed by MC Freda, EdD, RN, CHES, FAAN.

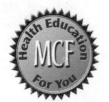

Woman's name: _____
Date: _____
Nurse's name: _____

Lunelle for Contraception

What is Lunelle?

Lunelle is a new birth control "shot." It is an injection of the same type of hormones that are in the birth control pill. The hormones are progesterone and estrogen. This method of contraception became available in October 2000, when the Food and Drug Administration approved its use.

How does it work???

Lunelle stops you from ovulating, so it prevents pregnancy. It has been shown to be 99% effective in preventing pregnancy. It is given by injection within the first 5 days of your period, or between 4 and 6 weeks after you have a baby. Then you get another injection every 28 to 30 days.

Why would you choose Lunelle?

Lunelle injections mean that you don't have to remember to take a birth control pill every day, and therefore you can't forget to take them. When you use Lunelle, you will have normal periods, and when you stop using it, you begin ovulating again within 2 to 4 months.

Is this different from the other birth control shot called Depo-Provera?

Yes, this is different, but it prevents pregnancy just as effectively. The Depo-Provera shot only has one hormone in it. The Depo-Provera shot is only given once every 3 months. With Depo-Provera, many women stop having periods after several injections. Some women like this, but this can make some women nervous about being pregnant. Another difference is that it can take up to a year for some women who stop the Depo-Provera shots to become pregnant.

Are there any side effects from Lunelle?

Yes, the side effects are the same as for the pill. Women who smoke, have high blood pressure, or a history of blood clots in the legs should not use this shot, or take the pill. Some women complain of weight gain, headaches, or breast tenderness.

   Remember that birth control shots and pills do not protect you from sexually transmitted diseases. Use condoms!

Flesch-Kincaid Reading Level: 7.0

Special Instructions _____

_____

Phone number to call if you have questions: _____

Copyright © Lippincott Williams & Wilkins. Developed by MC Freda, EdD, RN, CHES, FAAN.

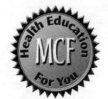

Woman's name: _____
Date: _____
Nurse's name: _____

El Anticonceptivo Lunelle

¿Qué es Lunelle?

Lunelle es una inyección nueva para el control de la natalidad. Es el mismo tipo de inyección de hormonas encontradas en las píldoras para el control de natalidad. Este método anticonceptivo apareció en el mercado en Octubre del año 2000 en el momento en que la Administración de Drogas y Alimentos aprobó su uso.

¿Cómo Funciona?

La Lunelle detiene la ovulación, previniendo así el embarazo. Se ha comprobado de que es 99 por ciento efectivo en la prevención del embarazo. Es aplicada mediante una inyección durante los primeros cinco días del periodo menstrual o dentro de 4 a 6 semanas después de tener a su bebé. Luego recibe otra inyección cada 28 a 30 días.

¿Por qué escogería Lunelle?

El uso de las inyecciones Lunelle significa de que no tiene que recordarse de tomar cada día las píldoras del control de natalidad y por consiguiente no se puede olvidar de tomarlas. Al usar Lunelle usted tendrá sus periodos de menstruación normales y cuando deje de usarla, usted comenzará a ovular nuevamente de 2 a 4 meses

¿Es Lunelle diferente a la otra inyección para el control de la natalidad llamada Depo-Provera?

Sí es diferente pero también efectiva para la prevención del embarazo. La inyección Depo-Provera contiene solamente una hormona y se aplica una vez cada 3 meses. Con la Depo-Provera y después de varias inyecciones, muchas mujeres paran de menstruar. Algunas mujeres le gusta este efecto, pero puede hacer nerviosas a otras pensando de que están embarazadas. Otra diferencia es que se puede tomar hasta un año para quedar embarazada después de parar las inyecciones de Depo-Provera.

¿Hay algún efecto secundario por la Lunelle?

Sí, los efectos secundarios son los mismos que los de la píldora. Las mujeres que fuman, tiene la presión alta, o con historial de coágulos de sangre en las piernas no deberían de usar esta inyección o tomar la píldora anticonceptiva. Algunas mujeres se quejan de aumento de peso, dolor de cabeza o senos adoloridos.

Recuerda que las inyecciones para el control de la natalidad y las píldoras anticonceptivas no le protejen de enfermedades venéreas. Use condones!!!!

Special Instructions _____

_____

Phone number to call if you have questions: _____

Copyright © Lippincott Williams & Wilkins. Developed by MC Freda, EdD, RN, CHES, FAAN.

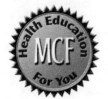

Woman's name: _____
Date: _____
Nurse's name: _____

The Diaphragm for Contraception

What is a diaphragm?

A diaphragm (pronounced "die-ah-fram") is a small piece of rubber shaped like the bottom of a cup. You put special cream or jelly in it, then you put the diaphragm in your vagina before you have sex. The cream kills some sperm, and the diaphragm keeps other sperm from getting to the egg. The diaphragm does not hurt you when it's inside you. It is about 80% effective at preventing pregnancy when you use it the right way every time you have sex. It looks like this:

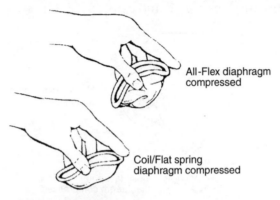

All-Flex diaphragm compressed

Coil/Flat spring diaphragm compressed

Why would you want to use a diaphragm?

If you don't want to take pills for birth control, or if you don't have sex very often, the diaphragm might be a good choice for you. You can put the diaphragm in your vagina up to 6 hours before you have sex. You should leave it in for 6 hours after you have sex. Because you can put it in a long time before sex, it does not interfere with sex. Your partner doesn't even have to know that you used it.

How do you get a diaphragm?

Your doctor, nurse, or midwife will give you a prescription for a diaphragm during your visit. You have to be measured to be sure you get the right size for you.

Are there side effects?

There are very few side effects. Most women have no problem with the diaphragm, but it does take time to learn how to put it in and take it out. Your doctor, nurse, or midwife will show you how to do it. Some women don't like touching themselves to put it inside and then take it out. If that's how you feel, then you might want to choose a different method of birth control.

Flesch-Kincaid Reading Level: 4.6

Special Instructions _____

_____

_____

Phone number to call if you have questions: _____

Copyright © Lippincott Williams & Wilkins. Developed by MC Freda, EdD, RN, CHES, FAAN.

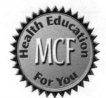

Health Education For You MCF

Woman's name: _____

Date: _____

Nurse's name: _____

El Diafragma como Anticonceptivo

¿Qué es un diafragma?

Un diafragma es una pequeña pieza de goma que tiene la forma del fondo de una taza. Usted le aplica una crema especial o gelatina , luego se coloca el diafragma dentro de su vagina antes de tener sexo. La crema mata algunos de los espermas, y el diafragma evita de que otros espermas lleguen hasta el huevo. Una vez dentro el diafragma no le causa dolor. Es como un ochenta por ciento efectivo en la prevención del embarazo cuando usted lo usa de la manera correcta;cada vez que tenga sexo. El diafragma luce algo como esto:

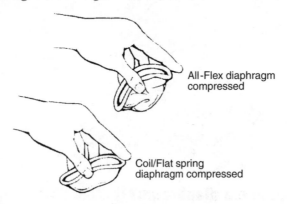

All-Flex diaphragm compressed

Coil/Flat spring diaphragm compressed

¿Por qué debería usted usar el diafragma?

Sí usted no desea tomar píldoras para el control de natalidad, o sí usted no tiene sexo muy a menudo el diafragma puede ser una buena selección para usted. Usted puede colocarse el diafragma dentro de su vagina hasta seis horas antes de tener sexo. Debería de dejarlo dentro por lo menos seis horas después de haber tenido sexo. Puesto de que usted se lo puede colocar mucho antes de tener relaciones sexuales ésto no interfiere con el sexo. Su pareja ni siquiera tiene que saber de que usted lo ha usado.

¿Cómo obtener un diafragma?

Su doctor, enfermera o comadrona le dara una prescripción para un diafragma durante su visita. Le tendran que tomar la medidas para asegurarse de que le den el tamaño correcto.

¿Existen efectos secundarios?

Existen muy pocos efectos secundarios. La mayoría de las mujeres no tienen problema con el diafragma, pero se toma tiempo en aprender cómo ponerlo y sacarlo. Su doctor, enfermera o comadrona le demostraran cómo hacerlo. Algunas mujeres no les gustan tocarse ellas mismas para ponérselo o sacárselo. Si usted se siente de ésta manera, debe de elegir un método diferente para el contro de la natalidad.

Special Instructions _____

_____

Phone number to call if you have questions: _____

Copyright © Lippincott Williams & Wilkins. Developed by MC Freda, EdD, RN, CHES, FAAN.

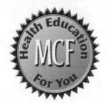

Woman's name: _____

Date: _____

Nurse's name: _____

The IUD for Contraception

What is an IUD?

IUD stands for "Intra-Uterine Device." It is a method of birth control (also called contraception) that can work for many years. It is very effective at preventing pregnancy (98%). It is a small T-shaped piece of plastic and copper that is placed inside your uterus by a doctor, nurse, or mid-wife. It has two strings at the end, which come out of your uterus into your vagina. You should check that the strings are there each month. The IUD looks something like this:

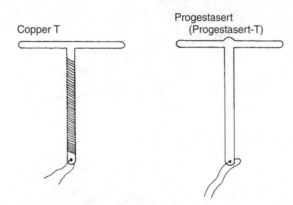

Why would you want an IUD for birth control?

An IUD can stay inside you for several years while it protects you from getting pregnant. You don't have to remember to take pills every day or to get shots. You don't have to put anything inside yourself (like a diaphragm or foam) each time you have sex. The IUD has medicine inside it that keeps the sperm from getting to the egg. The IUD is a good method of birth control for women who can't remember to take pills and for women who can't take the pills because of health problems like high blood pressure and blood clots. When you want to become pregnant, you have the IUD removed by a doctor, nurse, or midwife, and then you should be able to get pregnant.

Are there side effects to having an IUD?

Some women say that their periods are heavier when they have an IUD. A very small number of women might get an infection, but this is not common. If you are allergic to copper you might develop a rash. Remember that the IUD cannot protect you from sexually transmitted diseases.

Flesch-Kincaid Reading Level: 5.2

Special Instructions _____

_____

_____

_____

Phone number to call if you have questions: _____

Copyright © Lippincott Williams & Wilkins. Developed by MC Freda, EdD, RN, CHES, FAAN.

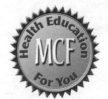

Woman's name: _____
Date: _____
Nurse's name: _____

El Dispositivo Intrauterino(DIU)
como Anticonceptivo

¿Qué es un DIU?

DIU quiere decir "Dispositivo Intrauterino." Es un forma del control de la natalidad (también llamado anticonceptivo) el cuál puede trabajar por muchos años. Es muy efectivo en la prevención de los embarazos (98 por ciento). Es una pequeña pieza de plástico y cobre en forma de T y es colocada dentro de su útero por un doctor, enfermera o comadrona. Al final tiene dos cuerdas que salen de su útero a su vagina. Cada més usted debe de chequear de que las cuerdas se encuentren allí. El DIU luce algo como ésto:

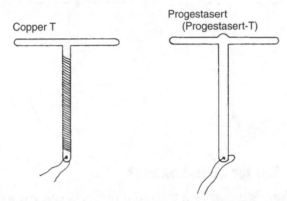

Copper T

Progestasert
(Progestasert-T)

¿Por qué quisiera usar un DIU para el control de la natalidad?

Un DIU puede permanecer dentro por muchos años mientras que la cuida de no salir embarazada. No tiene que recordarse de tomar las píldoras todos los días o que la inyecten. Usted no tiene que ponerse nada adentro(como un diafragma) cada vez que tenga sexo. El DIU tiene por dentro una medicina que previene que el esperma llegue al huevo. El DIU es un buen método del control de la natalidad para aquellas mujeres que no se pueden recordar de tomar las píldoras y para aquellas mujeres que no pueden tomar las píldoras debido a problemas de salud tales como la presión alta y coágulos de sangre. Cuando usted quiera salir embarazada, su DIU tiene que ser removido por un doctor, enfermera o comadrona y después usted podrá salir embarazada.

¿Hay efectos secundarios al tener un DIU?

Algunas mujeres dicen que sus reglas son más pesadas cuando tienen un DIU. Un número muy pequeño de mujeres pueden contraer una infección, más sin embargo ésto no es común. Sí usted es alérgica al cobre le puede desarrollar una erupción.

Special Instructions _____

_____

_____

Phone number to call if you have questions: _____

Copyright © Lippincott Williams & Wilkins. Developed by MC Freda, EdD, RN, CHES, FAAN.

Woman's name: _____

Date: _____

Nurse's name: _____

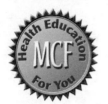

Natural Family Planning for Contraception

What Is Natural Family Planning?

Natural family planning (sometimes called the "rhythm" method or the "Fertility Awareness Method" [FAM]) is a way to practice birth control without using any pills or shots. When you use natural family planning, you find out when you are most likely to get pregnant, and then you do not have sex during that time.

How is Natural Family Planning done?

You must find out when you are ovulating, and then avoid sex (or use condoms) during that time. It is possible to become pregnant 2 days before you ovulate and then about 1 day after you ovulate. Most women ovulate between the 12th and 16th days of their cycle. Your menstrual cycle begins with the first day of your period. That means you probably ovulate 12 to 16 days after your period begins.

Before you can depend on natural family planning to avoid pregnancy, you must have a good understanding of your own body and your menstrual cycle. You should start keeping a record on paper of your periods and when you ovulate. Keep this record for about 6 months, so you can see how regular you are and how well you can predict when you are ovulating.

How Can You Tell When You Are Ovulating?

Some women have a mucus discharge from their vagina when they ovulate, but some don't. You can also take your temperature every morning before you get out of bed. Your temperature goes up a little bit when you ovulate. You can also buy an "ovulation kit" at the drug store, and that will tell you when you are ovulating.

Once you know when you usually ovulate, then you can plan when you will have sex. Most importantly, you can plan when you will not have sex. For most women, using natural family planning means that they do not have sex about 7 to 10 days in the middle of their cycle. The important thing is that they choose exactly the right days. This method of birth control has a failure rate of about 25%, so if you choose it, you should be prepared for what you will do if you become pregnant.

Talk to your doctor, nurse, midwife, or a trained natural family planning counselor about this. He or she can help you understand this method better and give you ideas about how it can work for you.

Flesch-Kincaid Reading Level: 7.4

Special Instructions _____

_____

Phone number to call if you have questions: _____

Copyright © Lippincott Williams & Wilkins. Developed by MC Freda, EdD, RN, CHES, FAAN.

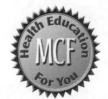

Woman's name: _____
Date: _____
Nurse's name: _____

Anticonceptivo Natural para la Planificación Familiar

¿Qué es la planificación natural familiar?

La planificación natural familiar (algunas veces denominada el método del "ritmo" o el "Método Conciente de Fertilización") es una manera de practicar el control de la natalidad sin utilizar ninguna píldoras o inyecciones. Cuando usted usa la planificación familiar natural, se entera cuando es más probable de salir embarazada, he aquí entonces de que durante éste tiempo no tenga relaciones sexuales.

¿Cómo se practica la planificación familiar natural?

Uste debe de averiguar cuando está ovulando, para luego evitar de tener sexo (o use condones) durante ése tiempo. Es posible salir embarazada dos días antes de que usted ovule y luego aproximadamente un día después de ovular. La mayoría de las mujeres ovulan entre el doceavo y el décimo sexto día de su ciclo. Su ciclo de menstruación empieza con el primer día de su regla. Probablemente eso quiere decir de que usted ovulará dentro de doce a dieciseis días después de que empieze su regla.

Antes de que usted empieze a depender de la planificación natural familiar para evitar el embarazo, usted debe tener un buen conocimiento de su cuerpo y de su ciclo menstrual. Usted debe de empezar a mantener por escrito un record de sus reglas y cuando ovula. Mantenga éste record aproximadamente por seis meses de tal manera de que pueda ver su regularidad y que tan bien puede predecir cuando está ovulando.

¿Cómo puede usted saber de que está ovulando?

Algunas mujeres cuando están ovulando, segregan de su vagina una mucosidad en cambio otras nó. Usted también puede tomarse la temperatura cada mañana antes de levantarse. Cuando usted ovula su temperatura le sube un poquito. Usted también puede comprar en la farmacia un "kit de ovulación" el cual le indicará cuando usted esté ovulando.

Una vez que usted sepa cuando generalmente ovula, puede planear cuando usted tendrá sexo. Lo más importante es de que usted puede planear cuando no desea tener sexo. Para la mayoría de las mujeres el uso de la planificación natural familiar significa el no tener sexo por siete días en la mitad de su ciclo. Lo importante es de que ellas escogen los siete días correctos. Este método del control de natalidad tiene un índice de error de aproximadamente un veinticinco por ciento (25%). Así de que si usted elige éste método usted debe de estar preparada para enfrentar la posibilidad de salir embarazada.

Hable con su doctor, enfermera o un consejero especializado acerca de ésto. Ellos le pueden ayudar a que comprenda mejor éste método y darle algunas ideas de como le puede funcionar a usted.

Special Instructions _____

_____

Phone number to call if you have questions: _____

Copyright © Lippincott Williams & Wilkins. Developed by MC Freda, EdD, RN, CHES, FAAN.

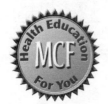

Spoiling and Other Myths About New Babies

Sometimes your mother or grandmother tells you things they learned about taking care of babies. Sometimes they are right, but sometimes the things they tell you are not right. There are some things about taking care of a new baby that have changed since your mother and grandmother had babies. Now that you are having a baby, it will be up to you to be sure that you understand what is right for taking care of a baby today, in the 21st century.

A myth is a saying or a story that people tell us but isn't really true. Here are some myths about taking care of new babies, compared with the real truth:

Myth: A baby should be fed every 4 hours, on a schedule.

Truth: A new baby should be fed whenever he or she is hungry, even if that is every 2 hours. Breast-fed babies often feed every 1 to 2 hours. If a newborn baby sleeps for more than 5 hours during the day (whether breast- or bottle-fed), you should wake the baby for feeding.

Myth: You will spoil a baby by picking her up whenever she cries.

Truth: Newborn babies need a lot of cuddling and holding, even when they are not being fed. You can't spoil a baby by holding and cuddling. You will just be showing your baby how much you love her.

Myth: All babies should be put to sleep on their stomachs.

Truth: All babies should be put to sleep on their backs. We now know that this can prevent Sudden Infant Death Syndrome (SIDS). There is a handout about this in this book.

Myth: Cereal in a baby's formula helps the baby sleep.

Truth: Babies do not need cereal right away. Talk to your doctor or nurse about this.

Myth: New babies should not go out of the house for 6 weeks.

Truth: It's good to protect babies from germs, but that doesn't mean the baby has to stay indoors for 6 weeks. Take the baby out when you feel well enough to go out.

Be sure to ask your doctor, nurse, or midwife about anything you want to know about taking care of your new baby.

Flesch-Kincaid Reading Level: 3.4

Special Instructions _____

_____

_____

Phone number to call if you have questions: _____

Copyright © Lippincott Williams & Wilkins. Developed by MC Freda, EdD, RN, CHES, FAAN.

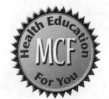

Woman's name: _____

Date: _____

Nurse's name: _____

Malcriadez y Otros Mitos Sobre los Recién Nacidos

Algunas veces tu mamá o abuela te comentaron cosas que ellas han aprendido sobre el cuidado del bebé. Muchas veces estan correctas en lo que dicen pero otras veces no lo estan. Hay muchos datos sobre cuidado del bebé que han cambiado desde que tu mamá ó tu abuela tuvieron niños. Ahora que vas a tener un bebé, dependerá de ti el aprender todo lo necesario sobre el cuidado de un recién nacido, especialmente ahora en el siglo 21.

Un mito es un dicho o historia que las personas dicen y por lo general no es verdad. He aquí algunos de los mitos sobre el cuidado de los recién nacidos:

Mito: Un bebé debe ser alimentado cada 4 horas, por reloj.

Verdad: Un recién nacido debe ser alimentado cuando sienta hambre, así fuera cada 2 horas. Los niños que toman el pecho, se alimentan cada 1 a 2 horas. Si el recién nacido duerme más de 5 horas durante el día (sea que tome biberón o el pecho) Usted debe despertarlo para que se alimente.

Mito: Vas a malcriar a tu bebé, si cada vez que llora lo recojes en tus brazos.

Verdad: Los recién nacidos necesitan mucha atención, amor y abrazos, aún cuando no están siendo alimentados. Usted no va a malcriar a su bebé por abrazarlo y mimarlo. Solo le estarás enseñando todo tu amor.

Mito: Todos los bebés deben ser puestos a dormir boca abajo.

Verdad: Todos los bebés deben ser puestos a dormir boca arriba, de espalda. Ahora sabemos que esto puede prevenir el Síndrome de Muerte Infantil.

Mito: El cereal en la formula ayudará a que tu bebé se duerma.

Verdad: Los bebés no necesitan cereal al principio. Hable con su doctor ó enfermera sobre esto.

Mito: Los recién nacidos no deben salir de la casa por 6 semanas.

Verdad: Es bueno proteger a los bebés contra los gérmenes, pero eso no quiere decir que tiene que permanecer en casa por 6 semanas. Saca a tu bebé de paseo solo cuando tu te sientas lo suficientemente bien como para hacerlo.

Asegúrate de preguntar a tu doctor, enfermera o comadrona sobre todo lo concerniente al cuidado de un bebé recién nacido.

Special Instructions _____

_____

_____

Phone number to call if you have questions: _____

Copyright © Lippincott Williams & Wilkins. Developed by MC Freda, EdD, RN, CHES, FAAN.

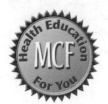

Woman's name: _____

Date: _____

Nurse's name: _____

Planning for Going Back to Work

Should you go back to work after having a baby?

No one can answer that question except you and your partner. It depends on many factors. Do you need the money? Do you have good child care? Do you want to go back to work? Would you rather be a stay-at-home-mother? It's a big decision, and you should take the time to think about all sides of the issue.

If you need to go back to work, when should you do it?

Most women find that at 6 to 8 weeks after giving birth they feel well enough to go back to work. Few women have more than 2 months of maternity leave, although some women are lucky enough to have 12 weeks of maternity leave. When you go back to work depends on your job, your family's needs, and your child care arrangements. Many women find they want to go back to work on a reduced schedule for a few months. Then they can get used to being away from the new baby gradually, and the baby can get used to the new caregiver.

Can you continue breast-feeding when you go back to work?

Even if you are not with your baby all day long, you can still breast-feed. Breast milk is the best food for a baby. You can pump your breasts and put the breast milk in a bottle for the caregiver to feed your baby while you're at work. During your workday, you can pump your breasts and keep the milk refrigerated. When you get home from work, you can breast-feed your baby normally.

Working and being a new mother can be very tiring. You don't get much sleep, and you have many responsibilities. Be sure that you ask for help from your partner, your family, or other people who love you. Be careful to eat a nutritious diet, drink a lot of water, and get as much sleep as you can so you will stay healthy.

Flesch-Kincaid Reading Level: 4.9

Special Instructions _____

_____

_____

_____

Phone number to call if you have questions: _____

Copyright © Lippincott Williams & Wilkins. Developed by MC Freda, EdD, RN, CHES, FAAN.

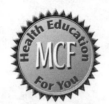

Woman's name: _____

Date: _____

Nurse's name: _____

Planeando el Regreso al Trabajo

¿Debería usted regresar a trabajar después de tener un bebé?

Nadie puede contestar ésta pregunta excepto usted y su pareja. Ello depende de muchos factores. ¿Necesita usted dinero? ¿Tiene usted un buen cuidado de niños? ¿Quiere usted regresar al trabajo? ¿Preferiría usted ser una madre que se queda en casa? Es una gran decisión y usted debe tomar su tiempo analizando todos los ángulos del caso.

¿Sí usted tiene necesidad de regresar a trabajar, cuándo debe de hacerlo?

La mayoría de las mujeres piensan de que pueden regresar a trabajar dentro de seis a ocho semanas después de haber dado a luz. Pocas mujeres toman una licencia por maternidad por más de dos meses, aunque algunas mujeres tienen la suficiente suerte de tener doce semanas de licencia por maternidad. El cuando regresar a trabajar depende de su trabajo, las necesidades familiars y los arreglos para el cuidado de su bebé. Muchas mujeres piensan en regresar a trabajar en un horario reducido por unos cuantos meses. Luego se pueden ir acostumbrando gradualmente a estar lejos de su nuevo bebé, y el bebé se pueda acostumbrar a su nuevo cuidador.

¿Puede usted continuar amamantando a su bebé cuando regrese a trabajar?

Aunque usted no esté con su bebé todo el día, todavía lo puede amamantar. La leche materna es la major comida para su bebé. Usted puede extraer leche de sus senos y poner la leche en una botella para que el cuidador alimente a su bebé mientras usted está en el trabajo. Usted puede extraer leche de sus senos durante sus horas de trabajo y mantener la leche refrigerada. Cuando llegue a casa después de trabajar usted puede normalmente amamantar a su bebé.

El trabajar y ser una nueva madre pueden ser muy fatigoso. Usted no puede dormir mucho y tiene muchas responsabilidades. Asegúrese de pedirle ayuda a su pareja, su familia u otras personas que la quieran. Tenga cuidado de comer dietas nutritivas, tomar mucha agua, y de dormir lo más que pueda, cosa de que se pueda mantener saludable.

Special Instructions _____

_____

_____

_____

Phone number to call if you have questions: _____

Copyright © Lippincott Williams & Wilkins. Developed by MC Freda, EdD, RN, CHES, FAAN.

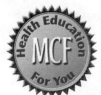

Woman's name: _____

Date: _____

Nurse's name: _____

Getting the Help You Need When You Go Home

You've had your baby. You're going home. Most women feel quite overwhelmed when they first go home with a new baby. You might have other children who need you, a house that needs cleaning, laundry that must be done, groceries to be bought, and, of course, you have a brand new baby to get to know and take care of. It can be very hard.

Asking for help

Many women feel they must do everything themselves. They can't seem to ask for help. They try to do everything, and then they become exhausted and can't do anything well. Don't fall into that trap. Now is the time to learn how to ask for help. If you have people who love you and are willing to help you, now is the time to talk to them. Don't be afraid to ask for help. Most women find that just getting their strength back and taking care of the baby is enough work for the first week they are home. So, ask the people who love you—perhaps it's your husband, your partner, your mother, your sister, your mother-in-law, or your good friend—to help with the rest of the things that need to be done in your life. Ask someone to watch your other children. Ask someone to shop for groceries and do your laundry. Ask someone to keep your kitchen clean or to take your other children to school or to after-school activities. Your only job that first week is then taking care of yourself and the new baby. Many women find that if they can just concentrate on the new baby and themselves for the first week, they recover from childbirth much quicker and feel better sooner.

Other things you can do

Your baby will probably be awake several times each night for feeding and changing, so you'll need to cope with that. Try to sleep while the baby is sleeping during the day. Turn the ringer off on your phone so it won't disturb your sleep. Get an answering machine to take messages so you can call people back when it's convenient for you. Ask your friends not to just "drop in" to see you, but to call first. Be sure to eat good nutritious food, and drink lots of water. Don't get overtired. Don't start exercising until your doctor, nurse, or midwife says it's okay. You body is still healing. Be sure to call your provider if you have heavy bleeding or severe pain anywhere or if you have a fever.

Soon you'll feel like yourself again. Enjoy quiet time with your new baby!

Flesch-Kincaid Reading Level: 4.3

Special Instructions _____

_____

_____

Phone number to call if you have questions: _____

Copyright © Lippincott Williams & Wilkins. Developed by MC Freda, EdD, RN, CHES, FAAN.

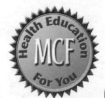
Como Obtener Ayuda Cuando Regresas a Casa

Tu bebé ha nacido. Los dos se marchan a casa. Muchas mujeres se sienten un poco desconcertadas al regresar a casa con un bebé recién nacido. Quizás tienes otros niños quienes te necesitan, una casa que necesita limpieza, lavar la ropa, hacer la compra de alimentos y por supuesto, un bebé nuevo a quien hay que conocer y cuidar. Es una situación un tanto difícil.

Pedir ayuda

Muchas mujeres piensan que lo tienen que hacer todo. Parecería que no quieren pedir ayuda. Tratan de hacerlo todo, llegando al agotamiento y luego no pueden hacer nada bien. No caigas en esta trampa. Ahora es el momento de aprender como pedir ayuda. Si tienes personas que te quieren y están dispuestas a ayudarte, ahora es el momento de hablarles. No tengas miedo de pedir ayuda. Muchas mujeres sienten que apenas se estan recuperando y el cuidado de un bebé es trabajo suficiente por las primeras semanas de regreso a casa. Así que pregunta a las personas que te quieren—quizás tu esposo, tu pareja, tu madre, tu hermana,tu suegra o tu mejor amiga—que te ayuden con el resto de los quehaceres del hogar. Pídele a alguien que te cuide los niños. Pídele a alguien que te compre la comida y te lave la ropa. Pídele a alguien que te mantega la cocina limpia, o que lleve los niños al colegio o a otras actividades después del colegio. Tu trabajo consistirá en cuidarte a tí misma y a tu bebé. Muchas mujeres piensan que si solamente se concentraran en ellas y en el cuidado del bebé por las primers semanas, ellos se recuperarían más rápido y se sentirían mejor.

Otras cosas que hacer

Tu bebé probablemente se despertará varias veces durante la noche para tomar su biberón y cambio de pañales. Tienes que enfrentar esa situación. Trata de dormir mientras que el bebé duerme durante el día. Apaga el timbre de teléfono así nadie te despertará y molestará tu descanso. Compra una máquina de mensajes, de ésta forma puedes contestar a toda aquellas personas que te llamaron. Pídele a tus amistades que no se presenten de improviso a visitarlos, pero que llamen primero. Asegúrate de comer saludable y nutritivo y toma mucha agua. No te excedas para no cansarte. No comiences a hacer ejercicios hasta que tu doctor, enfermera ó comadrona te lo permitan. Tu cuerpo todavía se está recuperando. Asegúrate de llamar a tu doctor, si tienes un periodo abundante ó dolor severo en cualquier lugar del cuerpo ó si tienes fiebre.

Pronto estarás como nueva. Disfruta tus momentos de tranquilidad junto a tu nuevo bebé!

Special Instructions _____

_____

Copyright © Lippincott Williams & Wilkins. Developed by MC Freda, EdD, RN, CHES, FAAN.

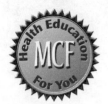

Woman's name: _____
Date: _____
Nurse's name: _____

Infant Care Assessment

After you have your baby, use this form to be sure that the nurses and midwives who care for you help you to learn what you need to know about newborn care.

Check the areas where you want to learn more before you go home with your baby, and show this to the nurses or midwives:

_____ How to breast-feed, how often to breast-feed

_____ How to decide if my breast-fed baby is getting enough milk

_____ How to take care of my breasts

_____ How to change a diaper

_____ How to take a baby's temperature

_____ How to know if the baby is sick and I should call the doctor or nurse

_____ How to take care of the baby's umbilical cord

_____ How and when to give the baby a bath

_____ Who to call if I have a question about the baby's health

_____ What to do if the baby won't stop crying

_____ Putting the baby to sleep—on his/her back or side?

_____ How to use the car seat

Flesch-Kincaid Reading Level: 4.4

Special Instructions _____

_____

_____

_____

_____

_____

Phone number to call if you have questions: _____

Copyright © Lippincott Williams & Wilkins. Developed by MC Freda, EdD, RN, CHES, FAAN.

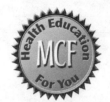

Woman's name: _____

Date: _____

Nurse's name: _____

Evaluación del Cuidado Infantil

Después de tener su bebé, use ésta página para estar segura de que las enfermeras y comadronas que cuidaron de usted, las ayuden a aprender lo que usted necesitará saber para cuidar a un recién nacido.

Antes de irse a su casa con su bebé, indique las áreas donde quiere aprender más y enséñeselo a las enfermeras o comadronas:

_____ Cómo y con qué frequencia amamantar

_____ Cómo determino si mi bebé que amamantó está recibiendo suficiente leche

_____ Cómo cuidar de mis senos

_____ Cómo cambiar un pañal

_____ Cómo tomar la temperatura de mi bebé

_____ Cómo sé si el bebé está enfermo y si debo llamar al doctor o a la enfermera

_____ Cómo cuidar del cordón umbilical del bebé

_____ Cómo y cuando debo bañar al bebé

_____ A quién debo llamar si tengo una pregunta sobre la salud del bebé

_____ Qué debo de hacer si mi bebé no para de llorar

_____ Donde dormirá el bebé y si debe de ser sobre su espalda o de costado

_____ Cómo usar el asiento del carro

Special Instructions _____

_____

_____

_____

_____

_____

_____

Phone number to call if you have questions: _____

Copyright © LIPPINCOTT WILLIAMS & WILKINS. Developed by MC Freda, EdD, RN, CHES, FAAN.

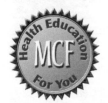

Woman's name: _____

Date: _____

Nurse's name: _____

Sometimes Things Go Wrong

No matter how much you want things to go well, even if you do everything you are supposed to do, sometimes things go wrong in a pregnancy or at a birth.

If your pregnancy ended with a less-than-perfect-outcome, you will probably need some help dealing with what happened. Sometimes babies are stillborn, and no one knows why. Sometimes babies are born with terrible health problems, which cause them to die shortly after birth. No one is ever prepared for such a tragedy. Remember that most times there wasn't anything you did to cause this.

There are some things that can be done to help you, and some organizations you will want to contact.

- If you had a miscarriage, you will need time to be sad and grieve for your loss. Sometimes this takes several months. You will need loving people around you to help you cope.
- If your baby was stillborn, or died shortly after birth, make sure that you spend some quiet time with your baby and your family. You need to see your baby, and you need to take as many pictures of your baby as you can. Be sure that your family brings a camera and lots of film to the hospital. Families whose newborn has died say that those pictures mean everything to them once they get home, because they are the only pictures they will ever have of their baby.
- If you are religious, you might want to talk to your priest, rabbi, or pastor.
- Call the March of Dimes at (888) MODIMES and ask for their bereavement packets. These written materials can be very helpful.
- Call RTS Bereavement Services (608) 785-0530 and ask for their booklet about babies who die.
- When you are ready, find a support group in your community to join. Compassionate Friends is one of these (www.compassionatefriends.org). Even though no one can feel exactly what you feel, other people who have lost infants can be very helpful to you.

Flesch-Kincaid Reading Level: 5.7

Special Instructions _____

_____

_____

_____

_____

Phone number to call if you have questions: _____

Copyright © Lippincott Williams & Wilkins. Developed by MC Freda, EdD, RN, CHES, FAAN.

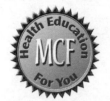

Woman's name: _____

Date: _____

Nurse's name: _____

Algunas Veces las Cosas Pueden Salir Mal

No importa lo mucho que usted quiera que las cosas salgan bién aún cuando usted hace todo al pie de la letra, algunas veces algo puede fallar en el embarazo o en el parto.

Si su embarazo terminó con un resultado no tan perfecto, probablemente usted necesitará alguna ayuda para enfrentar lo sucedido. Algunas veces los bebés nacen muertos y nadie sabe por qué. Algunas veces los bebés nacen con terribles problemas de salud lo que causa que mueran poco después de nacer. Nunca hay nadie preparado para enfrentar tal tragedia. Recuerde de que las mayoría de las veces nada de lo que usted hizo pudo haber causado ésto.

Existen algunas cosas que se pueden hacer para ayudarle y algunas organizaciones a las cuales usted querrá contactar.

- Si usted tuvo un aborto, necesitará tiempo para estar triste y afligida por su pérdida. Algunas veces ésto se toma muchos meses. Usted necesitará estar rodeada de gente cariñosa que la ayude a enfrentar la situación.
- Si su bebé nació muerto, o murió poco después de nacer, asegúrese de pasar unos momentos tranquilos con su bebé y su familia. Usted necesita ver a su bebé y necesita tomar la mayor cantidad posible de fotos. Esté segura de que su familia traiga una cámara al hospital. Aquellas familias a quienes sus recién nacidos han fallecido, dicen de que una vez que lleguen a casa aquellas fotos significan todo, ya que ésas serán las unicas fotos que tendrán de su bebé.
- Si usted es religiosa, usted debe de conversar con su sacerdote, rabino o pastor.
- Llame al March of Dimes al (888) 663-4637 y pida por sus paquetes de duelo. Estos materiales por escrito pueden ser muy útiles.
- Llame a los Servicios de Duelo RTS al (608) 785-0530 y solicite por su folleto sobre los bebés que han fallecido.
- Cuando usted esté lista, busque dentro de su comunidad un grupo de apoyo al cual se pueda unir. Uno de éstos es Amigos Compasionados (http:/www.compassionatefriends.org) Aunque nadie puede sentir exactamente lo que usted siente, otras personas que hayan perdido a sus infantes pueden ser de mucha ayuda para usted.

Special Instructions _____

_____

_____

_____

Phone number to call if you have questions: _____

Copyright © Lippincott Williams & Wilkins. Developed by MC Freda, EdD, RN, CHES, FAAN.

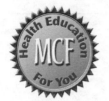

Woman's name: _____

Date: _____

Nurse's name: _____

Don't Forget Your Postpartum Visit . . .
It's Very Important!!!!

It is **very important** to see your doctor, nurse, or midwife for a "postpartum" check-up after your baby is born. Some providers ask you to come back at 2 weeks, or 4 weeks, or 6 weeks. At this visit your provider will:

- Examine you to make sure that your uterus and other organs have gone back to normal
- Help you choose a birth control method that is best for you
- Discuss how you are doing with the baby and anything else that you need to talk about

We advise you to wait to have sex until you are not having red bleeding anymore, until your stitches are healed (if you have any), and until you feel better. This is usually at least 2 weeks. Some women feel better waiting until after their postpartum check up to have sex again.

Remember that it is possible to become pregnant **as soon as you have sex for the first time** (even if you are breast-feeding), so **if you have sex be sure to use a condom.**

Congratulations—and we'll see you for your check-up!!!!

Flesch-Kincaid Reading Level: 7.9

Special Instructions _____

_____

_____

_____

_____

_____

_____

Phone number to call if you have questions: _____

Copyright © Lippincott Williams & Wilkins. Developed by MC Freda, EdD, RN, CHES, FAAN.

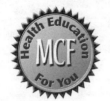

Woman's name: _____
Date: _____
Nurse's name: _____

No Olvide Su Visita Postpartum . . .
¡¡¡Es Muy Importante!!!

Es **muy importante** visitar a su doctor, enfermera o partera para un chequeo después que el bebé haya nacido. Algunos le pedirán que regrese a las 2 semanas, 4 semanas o 6 semanas. En esta visita su proveedor hará lo siguiente:

- Examinarla para estar seguro que su útero y otros órganos hayan regresado a lo normal
- Ayudarle a escojer el mejor método para prevenir el embarazo
- Discutir como está el bebé, y cualquier otra cosa de que quiera hablar

Le recomendamos no tener sexo mientras todavía esté sangrando, hasta que los puntos estén curados (si ha tenido algunos), y hasta que se sienta bien. Esto es por lo menos 2 semanas. Algunas mujeres esperan hasta después del chequeo para tener sexo nuevamente.

Recuerde que es posible quedar embarazada **desde la primera vez que tenga sexo** (a pesar que esté dando de pecho), por eso **si tiene sexo asegúrese de usar un condón.**

¡¡¡Felicitaciones—y la veremos en su próxima cita!!!

Special Instructions _____

_____

_____

_____

_____

_____

_____

Phone number to call if you have questions: _____

Copyright © Lippincott Williams & Wilkins. Developed by MC Freda, EdD, RN, CHES, FAAN.

216

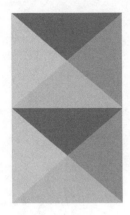

chapter 12

Interconceptional/
Preconceptional Care

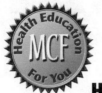

Woman's name: _____

Date: _____

Nurse's name: _____

How to Decide When to Become Pregnant Again

Did you know that having babies very close together can put you at risk for more health problems? Research has shown that if a woman has pregnancies closer than 18 months apart, she is more likely to have a baby with low birth weight. We now know that it takes your body about 1½ years to go completely back to normal after a pregnancy, and if you become pregnant before that, your body has to work extra hard.

So, it's a good idea to wait until your baby is about 18 months old before you try to become pregnant again, both for your health and for the health of the new baby. During that 18 months, be sure that you are taking 400 micrograms of Folic Acid every day either in a Folic Acid pill or in a multivitamin—that can prevent some forms of birth defects in your next pregnancy.

In addition to waiting 18 months, there are many things to consider when making the decision to become pregnant again:

- Your age and your partner's age
- Your finances
- Your health and your partner's health
- Your work situation
- The ages of your other children
- The desire of your partner to have more children

This is an important topic to mention to your doctor, your nurse, or your midwife. Be sure to make an appointment to see your provider, and discuss your plans for your next pregnancy. Planning your pregnancy can help you and your baby be healthy!

Flesch-Kincaid Reading Level: 6.7

Special Instructions _____

_____

_____

_____

_____

_____

Phone number to call if you have questions: _____

Copyright © Lippincott Williams & Wilkins. Developed by MC Freda, EdD, RN, CHES, FAAN.

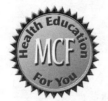

Woman's name: _____
Date: _____
Nurse's name: _____

Cuando Quedar Embarazada de Nuevo

¿Sabías que el quedar embarazada sin esperar un tiempo recomendable puede alzar el riesgo de problemas de salud? Estudios han confirmado que si los embarazos de una mujer son entre los primeros 18 meses, podrían correr el riesgo de un bebé con poco peso al nacer. Sabemos que tu cuerpo toma alrededor de un año a año y medio en volver a la normalidad después de un embarazo, y si quedas embarazada otra vez antes de ese período, tu cuerpo tiene que trabajar doblemente.

Así, que es una buena idea que esperes hasta que tu bebé tenga por lo menos 18 meses antes que trates de quedar embarazada otra vez, por tu salud y por la salud de tu nuevo bebé. Durante esos 18 meses, asegúrate de tomar 400 microgramos de ácido fólico todos los días, sea en forma de multivamina o en píldora-esto puede prevenir algunas formas de defectos congénitos en tu próximo embarazo.

Además de esperar los 18 meses, existen otros puntos a considerar cuando tomes ésta decisión:

- Tu edad y la edad de tu pareja.
- Tu situación económica.
- Tu salud y la salud de tu pareja.
- Tu situación laboral
- Las edades de tus otros hijos(as)
- El deseo de tu pareja de tener o no más hijos(as)

Este es un tópico muy importante que debes mencionar a tu doctor, enfermera o comadrona. Asegúrate de hacer una cita con tu doctor, y explicarle tus planes acerca de la posibilidad de un nuevo embarazo. ¡El planear cuidadosamente un embarazo puede ser muy beneficioso para tí y para un bebé saludable!

Special Instructions _____

_____

_____

_____

_____

Phone number to call if you have questions: _____

Copyright © Lippincott Williams & Wilkins. Developed by MC Freda, EdD, RN, CHES, FAAN.

Woman's name: _____

Date: _____

Nurse's name: _____

What Can You Do to Protect Your Next Baby From Birth Defects?

Birth defects, such as Spina Bifida, can be very difficult for both parents and the affected children. Spina bifida (also called a "neural tube defect") means that during pregnancy, the spinal cord of the growing fetus doesn't get covered by muscle and skin as it should, and some of it stays exposed. There are several different types of spina bifida, from very mild to very severe. In many cases the child with spina bifida will never be able to walk and may have bowel and bladder problems.

But something wonderful has happened recently. We have learned that there is something women can do to help prevent many cases of spina bifida. It's a very simple thing, and very easy to do. It's just taking a vitamin called Folic Acid (Folic Acid is one of the B vitamins) every day before becoming pregnant, and early in pregnancy. It's that simple.

Before you plan to become pregnant again, start taking 400 micrograms (mcg) of Folic Acid every day. You don't need a prescription. That is the usual dose in a regular multivitamin, but you should read the label or ask the pharmacist to be sure that the vitamin bottle you buy has 400 mcg of Folic Acid in every pill. If the pill you buy doesn't have 400 mcg of Folic Acid in it, don't take two vitamin pills to get the 400 mcg. Then you might be getting too much of another vitamin. Ask the pharmacist for a vitamin that has 400 mcg of Folic Acid in it. As a matter of fact, you should start taking that pill every day, starting right now. Why? Because many women become pregnant even when they didn't plan to become pregnant, and there's no sense in taking a chance.

You must be taking the folic acid before the pregnancy for it to work to prevent spina bifida. So start taking it every day! Start now!!!

Flesch-Kincaid Reading Level: 7.6

Special Instructions _____

_____

_____

_____

_____

_____

Phone number to call if you have questions: _____

Copyright © Lippincott Williams & Wilkins. Developed by MC Freda, EdD, RN, CHES, FAAN.

Health Education For You — MCF

Woman's name: _____

Date: _____

Nurse's name: _____

¿Qué Puede Hacer Usted Para Proteger A Su Bebé De Defectos Congénitos?

Los defectos congénitos (adquiridos durante el desarrollo del feto) como Espina Bífida puede ser muy difícil tanto como para los padres como para el niño(a) que los sufre. Espina Bífida (también conocida como defecto del tubo neural) significa que durante el embarazo, la médula espinal del feto no se cubre con músculo y piel como debería hacerlo, entonces una sección de la médula queda expuesta. Hay diferentes tipos de Espina Bífida, desde la más leve hasta la más severa. En muchos casos el niño(a) con Espina Bífida nunca podrá caminar, y podría tener problemas de defecación y de orinar.

Pero algo maravilloso ha pasado recientemente . Hemos aprendido que hay algo que la mujeres embarazadas pueden hacer para evitar muchos casos de espina bífida. Es una cosa muy sencilla, y fácil de hacer. Se trata de tomar una vitamina llamada Acido Fólico (Acido fólico es una forma de la vitamina B) todos los días antes te salir en estado, y durante el primer trimestre del embarazo. Es así de simple.

Antes de que planees salir en estado otra vez, comienza a tomar 400 microgramos (mcg) de ácido fólico todos los días. No necesitas receta médica. Esta es una dósis normal en un complejo multivitamínico, pero debes leer la etiqueta, o pregunta a tu farmacista para asergurarte que la botella de vitamina que estas comprando contiene 400 mcg de ácido fólico en cada píldora. Si las píldoras que comprastes no contienen 400 mcg de áido fóico, no tienes que tomar dos pastillas para obtener los 400mcg. Estarías consumiendo el doble de las dósis ndicada para las otras vitaminas. Pregúntale a tu farmacista por unas vitaminas que contengan ácido fólico. A próposito, deberías de comenzar a tomar esa pastilla todos los días, comenzando ahora. ¿Por qué? Porque muchas mujeres quedan embarazadas aún cuando no esten haciendo planes de hacerlo, por lo que no hay que correr ningun riesgo.

Debes tomar Acido Fólico antes del embarazo para que ello comienze a trabajar y prevenir la espina bífida. Así que comienza a tomarla ahora. ¡Comienza yá!!!

Special Instructions _____

_____

_____

_____

Phone number to call if you have questions: _____

Copyright © Lippincott Williams & Wilkins. Developed by MC Freda, EdD, RN, CHES, FAAN.

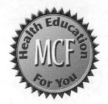

Woman's name: _____

Date: _____

Nurse's name: _____

Emergency Contraception

What is emergency contraception?

Emergency contraception is what some people call "the morning after pill," but it is used longer than just the next day. It should never be used as your regular method of birth control. It is just for emergencies such as:

• If you had unprotected sex
• If the condom broke
• If you find out your partner did not wear a condom
• If you were raped

   If any of those things happen, you can take a special combination of birth control pills to keep from becoming pregnant. It works by either keeping the egg from being released from the ovary, or slowing the movement of the egg into the tube, or keeping a fertilized egg from implanting in the uterus. This method is about 75% effective at preventing pregnancy.

How many pills do you take?

If you have birth control pills at home, you should call your doctor, nurse, or midwife and tell him or her that you want to use the pills for emergency contraception. If you cannot reach anyone right away, then you should take two pills as soon as possible. Keep trying to call your provider. He or she will tell you to take two more pills 12 hours later. The longest you can wait to take the first 2 pills is 3 days after the unprotected sex. If you do not have birth control pills at home, you should immediately call your health care provider and get a prescription. You should tell the doctor, nurse, or midwife why you need the prescription so quickly. If you wait past the 3 days after unprotected sex to take the emergency contraception, it might not work.

Are there side effects?

Yes, many women who use emergency contraception have nausea and vomiting. Some have headaches also. Most of the side effects go away in a few days.

   Emergency contraception should only be used in real emergencies. If you need to use it, take that opportunity to talk to your provider about a method of birth control that you can depend on every day. Remember that only condoms can protect you from sexually transmitted diseases and HIV.

Flesch-Kincaid Reading Level:6.4

Special Instructions _____

_____

Phone number to call if you have questions: _____

Copyright © Lippincott Williams & Wilkins. Developed by MC Freda, EdD, RN, CHES, FAAN.

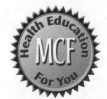

Anticonceptivos de Emergencia

¿Qué es un anticonceptivo de emergencia?

El anticonceptivo de emergencia es lo que algunas personas denominan "la píldora mañanera", aunque sólo puede ser usada más que solamente el día siguiente. Ella nunca debe de ser usada como un método para el control de la natalidad. Se usa sólo para casos de emergencias tales como:

- Si ha tenido sexo sin protección
- Si el condón se rompió
- Si se entera que su pareja no usó un condón
- Si usted fué violada

Si sucede algunas de éstas cosas, usted puede tomar una combinación especial de píldoras anticonceptivas para prevenir de quedar en estado. Ella funciona evitando de que el huevo sea liberado del ovario o disminuyendo el movimiento del huevo dentro de la trompa, o evitando de que un huevo fertilizado se implante dentro del útero. Este método es setenta y cinco por ciento (75%) efectivo en prevenir los embarazos.

¿Cuántas píldoras debe usted tomar?

Si usted tiene píldoras anticonceptivas en su casa, debería de llamar a su doctor, enfermera o comadrona y decirles de que desea usar las píldoras como anticonceptivos de emergencia. Si usted no puede comunicarse con nadie al instante, debería luego tomarse dos píldoras tan pronto le sea posible. Sigua insistiendo en llamar a su proveedor. Ellos le dirán de que tome dos píldoras más, doce horas más tarde.Lo más que usted puede esperar para tomar las primeras dos píldoras es tres días después de haber tenido sexo sin protección. Si usted no tiene en su casa las píldoras anticoceptivas, inmediatamente debería de llamar a su proveedor de servicios médicos y obtener una prescripción. Debería de decirle a su doctor, enfermera o comadrona el por qué usted necesita las píldoras tan rápido. Si usted espera que pasen más de tres días después de haber tenido sexo sin protección, pueda de que las píldoras no trabajen.

¿Existen efectos secundarios?

Sí, muchas mujeres que usan el anticonceptivo de emergencia les da náusea y vómitos. A algunas les dá dolores de cabeza. La mayoría de los efectos secundarios desaparecen en pocos días.

Los anticonceptivos de emergencia solamente deberían ser usados en casos de emergencias reales. Si usted necesita usarla aproveche ésa oportunidad para conversar con su doctor acerca de un método para el control de natalidad del cual usted pueda depender todos los días.Recuérdese de que solamente los condones lo protegen de enfermedades transmitidas sexualmente y del virus de inmunodeficiencia humana.

Special Instructions _____

_____

_____

Phone number to call if you have questions: _____

Copyright © Lippincott Williams & Wilkins. Developed by MC Freda, EdD, RN, CHES, FAAN.

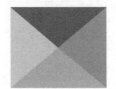

Index

Page references followed by the letter *b* indicate information located in a box. Page references followed by the letter *f* indicate illustrative material.

PROGRAM LICENSE AGREEMENT

Read carefully the following terms and conditions before using the Software. Use of the Software indicates your and, if applicable, your Institution's acceptance of the terms and conditions of this License Agreement.

If you do not agree with the terms and conditions, you should promptly return this package to the place you purchased it and your payment will be refunded.

Definitions

As used herein, the following terms shall have the following meanings:

"Software" means the software program contained on the diskette(s) or CD-ROM or preloaded on a workstation and the user documentation, which includes all accompanying printed material.

"Institution" means a nursing or professional school, a single academic organization that does not provide patient care and is located in a single city and has one geographic location/address.

"Geographic location" means a facility at a specific location; geographic locations do not provide for satellite or remote locations that are considered a separate facility.

"Facility" means a health care facility at a specific location that provides patient care and is located in a single city and has one geographic location/address.

"Publisher" means Lippincott Williams & Wilkins, Inc., with its principal office in Philadelphia, Pennsylvania.

"Developer" means the company responsible for developing the software as noted on the product.

License

You are hereby granted a nonexclusive license to use the Software in the United States. This license is not transferable and does not authorize resale or sublicensing without the written approval or an authorized officer of Publisher.

The Publisher retains all rights and title to all copyrights, patents, trademarks, trade secrets, and other proprietary rights in the Software. You may not remove or obscure the copyright notices in or on the Software. You agree to use reasonable efforts to protect the Software from unauthorized use, reproduction, distribution, or publication.

Single-User license

If you purchased this Software program at the Single-User License price or a discount of that price, you may use this program on one single-user computer. You may not use the Software in a time-sharing environment or otherwise to provide multiple, simultaneous access. You may not provide or permit access to this program to anyone other than yourself.

Institutional/Facility license

If you purchased the Software at the Institutional or Facility License Price or at a discount of that price, you have purchased the Software for use within your Institution/Facility on a single workstation/computer. You may not provide copies of or remote access to the Software. You may not modify or translate the program or related documentation. You agree to instruct the individuals in your Institution/Facility who will have access to the Software to abide by the terms of this License Agreement. If you or any member of your Institution fail to comply with any of the terms of this License Agreement, this license shall terminate automatically.

Network license

If you purchased the Software at the Network License Price, you may copy the Software for use within your Institution/Facility on an unlimited number of computers within one geographic location/address. You may not provide remote access to the Software over a value-added network or otherwise. You may not provide copies of or remote access to the Software to individuals or entities who are not members of your Institution/Facility. You may not modify or translate the program or related documentation. You agree to instruct the individuals in your Institution/Facility who will have access to the Software to abide by the terms of this License Agreement. If you or any member of your Institution/Facility fail to comply with any of the terms of this License Agreement, this license shall terminate automatically.

Limited warranty

The Publisher warrants that the media on which the Software is furnished shall be free from defects in materials and workmanship under normal use for a period of 90 days from the date of delivery to you, as evidenced by your receipt of purchase.

The Software is sold on a 30-day trial basis. If, for whatever reason, you decide not to keep the software, you may return it for a full refund within 30 days of the invoice date or purchase, as evidenced by your receipt of purchase by returning all parts of the Software and packaging in saleable condition with the original invoice, to the place you purchased it. If the Software is not returned in such condition, you will not be entitled to a refund. When returning the Software, we suggest that you insure all packages for their retail value and mail them by a traceable method.

The Software is a computer assisted instruction (CAI) program that is not intended to provide medical consultation regarding the diagnosis or treatment of any specific patient.

The Software is provided without warranty of any kind, either expressed or implied, including but not limited to any implied warranty of fitness for a particular purpose of merchantability. Neither Publisher nor Developer warrants that the Software will satisfy your requirements or that the Software is free of program or content errors. Neither Publisher nor Developer warrants, guarantees, or makes any representation regarding the use of the Software in terms of accuracy, reliability or completeness, and you rely on the content of the programs solely at your own risk.

The Publisher is not responsible (as a matter of products liability, negligence, or otherwise) for any injury resulting from any material contained herein. This Software contains information relating to general principles of patient care that should not be construed as specific instructions for individual patients.

Manufacturers' product information and package inserts should be reviewed for current information, including contraindications, dosages, and precautions.

Some states do not allow the exclusion of implied warranties, so the above exclusion may not apply to you. This warranty gives you specific legal rights and you may also have other rights that vary from state to state.

Limitation of remedies

The entire liability of Publisher and Developer and your exclusive remedy shall be: (1) the replacement of any CD which does not meet the limited warranty stated above which is returned to the place you purchased it with your purchase receipt; or (2) if the Publisher or the wholesaler or retailer from whom you purchased the Software is unable to deliver a replacement CD free from defects in material and workmanship, you may terminate this License Agreement by returning the CD, and your money will be refunded.

In no event will Publisher or Developer be liable for any damages, including any damages for personal injury, lost profits, lost savings or other incidental or consequential damages arising out of the use or inability to use the Software or any error or defect in the Software, whether in the database or in the programming, even if the Publisher, Developer, or an authorized wholesaler or retailer has been advised of the possibility of such damage.

Some states do not allow the limitation or exclusion of liability for incidental or consequential damages. The above limitations and exclusions may not apply to you.

General

This License Agreement shall be governed by the laws of the State of Pennsylvania without reference to the conflict of laws provisions thereof, and may only be modified in a written statement signed by an authorized officer of the Publisher. By opening and using the Software, you acknowledge that you have read this License Agreement, understand it, and agree to be bound by its terms and conditions. You further agree that it is a complete and exclusive statement of the agreement between the Institution/Facility and the Publisher, which supersedes any proposal or prior agreement, oral or written, and any other communication between you and Publisher or Developer relative to the subject matter of the License Agreement.

Note
Attach a paid invoice to the License Agreement as proof of purchase.

Minimum System Requirements

- a Pentium 100 CPU;
- 32 MB RAM (64 recommended);
- Windows;
- SVGA display supporting 256 colors (16 bit recommended);
- 12X CD-ROM drive;
- 800x600 monitor resolution;
- mouse;
- 5 MB of hard-disk space

Note

In order to view the PDF files, you must have Adobe Acrobat Reader installed on your PC. If you do not currently have this program installed, it is a free download available at: http://www.adobe.com/products/acrobat/read-step.html

Running the program

The program should automatically start a few seconds after you have inserted the CD-ROM into your CD-ROM drive. If the program does not automatically start, follow these steps:

1. Open the Start menu and select Run.
2. In Open box, type d:\PerinatalPatientForms.html, where d is the letter representing your CD-ROM drive, and press Enter. (If your CD-ROM drive is a letter other than d, substitute that letter.)
3. Double-click on the PerinatalPatient file to launch the program.